WITHDRAWN

A Woman's Guide to Sleep

A Woman's *Guide to* Sleep

GUARANTEED SOLUTIONS FOR A GOOD NIGHT'S REST

Joyce A. Walsleben, Ph.D.,
Director of the Sleep Disorders Center
at New York University School of Medicine

Rita Baron-Faust

CROWN PUBLISHERS

NEW YORK

Published by Crown Publishers, New York, New York.
Member of the Crown Publishing Group.

Random House, Inc., New York, Toronto, London, Sydney, Auckland
www.randomhouse.com

CROWN is a trademark and the Crown colophon is a
registered trademark of Random House, Inc.

Printed in the United States of America
Design by Ann Gold

Library of Congress Cataloging-in-Publication Data
Walsleben, Joyce A.
A woman's guide to sleep : guaranteed solutions for a good night's rest /
Joyce A. Walsleben and Rita Baron-Faust.—1st ed.
p.   cm.
Published simultaneously in Canada by Random House of Canada Limited, Toronto.
Includes bibliographical references and index.
1. Insomnia—Treatment. 2. Women—Health and hygiene.
3. Sleep—Physiological aspects. 4. Sleep disorders—Treatment.
I. Baron-Faust, Rita. II. Title.
RC548.W35   2000
612.8'21'082—dc21   00-027999

ISBN 0-8129-3259-5
10 9 8 7 6 5 4 3 2 1
First Edition

*To all the wonderful women in my life whose support and love has fed me and
    especially*

*My mother, Alice Cornelius, friends Ruth Nelson and Ruth Baum, who do so
    now in spirit.*

*The "Group": Cathy Simpson, Jeanette Kraus, Estelle Herskovitz, Nena O'Neil,
    and Jane Porcino.*

*My own: daughter Linda, daughter-in-law Carolynn, Chris, and the special lady
    of the future, granddaughter Kersten Elizabeth!*

JAW

To all those who have encouraged and supported me:

My husband, Allen, who has shown me how love weathers the storms

*My son, Alexander, I hope I've set an example he'll want to follow in
    whatever work he chooses*

*My mother, who has inspired me with her strength to overcome loss
    and to cope with knee surgery much better than I ever could*

*And to my aunt, Eleanor Berman, who helped steer me on a realistic course
    when I embarked on my journey as a writer*

RBF

Author's Note

No book, including this one, can substitute for the personal care of your doctor. I hope you'll use this book to work more effectively with your doctor to resolve your sleep concerns. Let me reiterate here that you should never take any medication or supplement without informing your doctor. Please do share this book with your health care team. I wish you pleasant dreams.

Acknowledgments

It is important to know that while this book is based on my experience as a clinician, its basis is formed from the work of others in the field, and we all owe them our thanks. The field is relatively young, with most of the fathers (and mothers) still alive and actively working. They have all shared their work eagerly over the years and continue to do so. Throughout the book I have referenced their work and noted in Appendix III what sources could be helpful to the reader. Please explore further as your interest dictates. The work has been supported in a number of ways, from federal funding to private foundation monies. We owe our thanks to these agencies and the tireless researchers who explore.

I especially want to thank my original mentors, Drs. Nancy K. Squires, Merrill M. Mitler, and Richard Allen, for the excitement they shared and their ongoing support. I am deeply indebted to my colleagues at NYU, Drs. Roberta Goldring and David Rapoport, for giving me the opportunity to establish the clinical laboratory and particularly for their patience in the frenzy of writing this book. Additional recognition goes to the current staff of the center, who are always so supportive, as well as my past students Drs. Elise Caccappolo and Rochelle Zozula for funneling me the very latest information related to sleep and women.

A special thank-you to my coauthor, Rita Baron-Faust, for taking the chance, for sharing her wonderful ability to write and her extensive knowledge regarding women's health issues. Get some sleep, Rita! A huge thank-you to our agent, Vicky Bijur, who believed in the concept and really supported us throughout this endeavor. And finally to our editor, Betsy Rapoport, whose humor, probing questions, and patience made this possible.

Fortunately, this book is not the final word on sleep in women. Exciting research continues in both humans and animals, on both behavioral and molecular levels. As researchers we need your help. I ask you to recognize the need and value of this research. Please support its concept and funding in whatever way you can and join in when possible. We can work together to improve awareness of and comfort regarding sleep and its consequences.

JAW

This book began with a routine interview. I have known Dr. Joyce Walsleben for many years. We were in the midst of a radio interview on sleep and aging when she mentioned that she had often thought of doing a book about women's sleep issues. I said it sounded like a great idea. That meeting began a wonderful partnership and friendship.

I'm deeply grateful to Joyce for the chance to work with her on this groundbreaking book. It's my first partnership on a book, and I've learned a great deal. Plus, we had lots of fun.

I am also grateful to my agent, Vicky Bijur, who enthusiastically supported my four previous books, and who embraced this project as well.

Our editor, Betsy Rapoport, was a delight to work with and a source of many questions and much shared humor. We are so happy that she shared our vision.

I am thankful that my husband, Allen, who must rise early in the morning for his work as a television news producer, has been so understanding about my many late nights writing this book. His support is my bedrock. My son, Alexander, has been a source of pride and joy as he navigates his middle school years (and negotiates a later bedtime). And thanks go to my mother, who has always been my best editor, for her continued support, encouragement, and love. Now maybe *I* can get some sleep!

RBF

Contents

Introduction

Women are probably the most sleep-deprived creatures on earth.

The average woman aged thirty to sixty sleeps only six hours and forty-one minutes a night during the workweek; most people need at least eight hours of sleep to function at their best.

The irony is, women actually have an *advantage* when it comes to the structure of their sleep. It may not seem like it on most nights, but sleep laboratory studies show that women have more deep, restorative sleep than men. We tend to sleep longer, wake up less often, and suffer less from certain sleep disorders. But all too often, life circumstances sabotage this natural advantage. And too many of us end up driving drowsy, working at half throttle, and trying to make up for lost sleep time on the weekends.

A landmark 1998 survey by the National Sleep Foundation found that conditions unique to females rob *56 percent of women* of a good night's sleep! (You'll be hearing more about the survey throughout the book.) Our sleep is disrupted by the hormonal surges of puberty, pregnancy, premenstrual syndrome, and perimenopause. Not to mention late nights caused by the competing demands of careers and children, the "second shift," and caring for a newborn (or an aging family member). In fact, a woman may lose as much as seven hundred hours of sleep during her baby's first year of life!

Then there's sex; men drift off to blissful sleep after lovemaking, while we're left wide awake.

Hot flashes interrupt sleep during the menopausal years. Of the 17 million Americans with overactive bladder, the vast majority are women, whose sleep is disrupted several times a night by trips to the bathroom. In older age our natural sleep-wake patterns change so that we may awaken before dawn. Our sleep may be shattered by the pain of arthritis or other chronic diseases more common in women.

As a result, 50 percent more women than men report that daytime sleepiness interferes with daily activities, 32 percent of women use sleep medications, compared with 21 percent of men, and nearly a quarter more women than men report insomnia a few nights a week. The only area where men report *more* problems: 66 percent admit to driving drowsy, compared with 49 percent of women.

It should be said that these kinds of surveys (which the National Sleep Foundation conducts every year) are not perfect. They are aimed at finding answers to specific questions, such as the number of people driving drowsy or using sleep aids. But they do provide a window into how well Americans are sleeping. And they also reveal how surprisingly little we know about this vital bodily function.

The foundation recently polled one thousand Americans about their knowledge of sleep, and if we applied the results to the general population, we'd find that an astounding 168 million adults believe myths about sleep that could be dangerous to their health. For example, most people believe that snoring is not a health problem. In fact, it can be a symptom of a disorder called obstructive sleep apnea (see page 133), which can be life-threatening. People also believe that turning up the volume on the car radio will keep you awake when you drive at night. But it's not true. If you're sleep-deprived, even a raucous heavy metal band won't keep you from nodding off.

Given all the factors that interfere with women's sleep, and our lack of knowledge about sleep, there's been precious little advice out there to help women get a better night's sleep. Textbooks on sleep medicine barely mention women, other than to discuss pregnancy or hot flashes. Most sleep studies have been done on men and the results applied to women. No wonder when women leaf through the dozens of how-to books on sleep they find little that's relevant to their lives, or the information is just too scientific to be useful.

Well, we're going to change all that.

For the first time, a sleep book is putting the emphasis on you. On us. On the hormonal, age-related, family, and social factors that too often conspire to deny us a good night's sleep.

In my twenty years' experience as a sleep researcher and clinician, I have helped many women solve their sleep problems. Most of the advice I give is a commonsense interpretation of research, rather than a technical discourse. More than a few patients have said to me, "You should write a book." So I did.

I have taken typical patient questions and sleep problems and responded to them, combining the knowledge we've gained in the sleep lab with practical ways to use it in your everyday life. Throughout the book you'll also find tips on what foods, beverages, herbs, and (when you need them) medications can help sleep. Some of the information I'll be giving you is very new and has never been gathered in one place before. Some of the research you'll be reading about is still evolving, so we have more questions than answers.

I've tried to make this a personal book, your own consultation with a sleep therapist. After reading it, you should have answers to many of your questions about sleep and, I hope, have gained some strategies for better sleep. And I hope you'll have learned things about sleep that may help your family members and loved ones, too.

I wish you happy reading and a wonderfully satisfying night's sleep.

A Woman's Guide to Sleep

1

How and Why We Sleep

Ways to Sleep Better

How many hours of sleep did you get last night? Five hours? Six?

You're not alone. The average woman gets barely six and a half hours of sleep most nights. During any given month more than *half* of the women surveyed report symptoms of insomnia. The National Sleep Foundation (NSF) Women and Sleep Poll found that lack of sleep interferes with the daily activities of at least three out of every ten women. Almost a third of us are using over-the-counter or prescription sleep aids at night, while 31 percent turn to caffeine and medications to combat daytime sleepiness. Worse, 6 percent are using alcohol as a sleep aid.

Why is this happening?

Women's sleep is affected by many factors: hormones, age, life situations, and problems that affect us in greater numbers than men, such as depression and pain syndromes. On top of that, most of us don't know enough about sleep . . . or how to get the best of it. So before we discuss the special sleep problems we face as women, let's look at how and why we sleep and go over some basic strategies for getting a better night's rest.

The Female Advantage?

The structure of women's sleep is fundamentally the same as men's, but there are some very positive differences.

For one thing, women have more *slow-wave sleep (SWS), also called stage 3 and 4 sleep,* the deepest, most restorative level of sleep. This difference turns up at around six months of age. After around ten months, baby girls tend to sleep more than boys. We have fewer arousals during the night. Boys, by contrast, have more periods of *rapid eye movement sleep (REM),* the main period during which we dream (more about the stages of sleep later on).

We hold on to this extra slow-wave sleep as we age. In fact, women's sleep systems seem to age at a slower pace than men's. Men start a deterioration of slow-wave sleep during their twenties, whereas in women the decline begins in our thirties and progresses more slowly. In fact, a fifty-something woman's sleep patterns are equivalent to those of a thirty-year-old man.

Now you ask: If I'm supposed to be sleeping so much better than a man, why am I so tired?

Our total sleep time gets less as we enter our forties and fifties. As we inch toward menopause, our number of sleep stage changes increases and we awake more during the night. This is probably the result of the hormonal and vasomotor changes of perimenopause and menopause, such as hot flashes.

In its survey on women and sleep, the NSF found that menopausal women experience hot flashes during sleep three days out of the week and have difficulty sleeping caused by hot flashes an average of five days per month. Even with that, women still experience more slow-wave sleep than men and have more total sleep time. In men, awakenings during the night and frequency of lighter sleep periods *(stage 1 sleep)* increase during the sixties.

During older age men and women both have fewer sleep stage shifts, and periods of deep sleep further decline in men. Our sleep patterns also shift slightly, making us feel more tired in the early evening and awakening us before dawn (I'll explain this on page 104). Also disturbing sleep for many of us in later life are bladder problems and pain from conditions such as arthritis.

All of this data on women's sleep comes from observing healthy, normal people in a quiet research environment. There are no crying babies, sick kids, snoring partners. In other words, real-life conditions can sab-

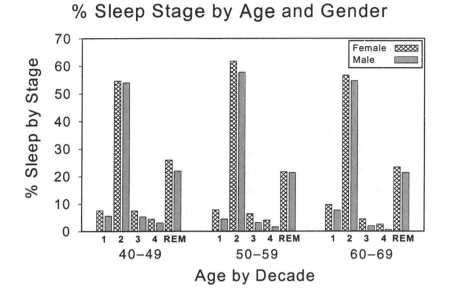

Men get less slow-wave sleep, and a little less dream sleep.

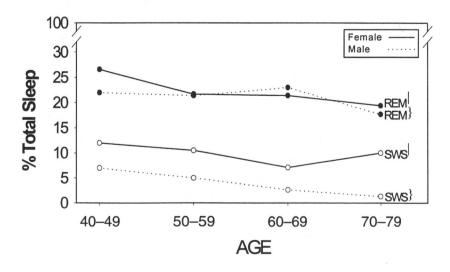

Women hold on to deep, restful sleep throughout
middle age and into older age.

otage those (technically) splendid female sleep patterns. But that doesn't mean you *can't* get a better night's sleep. We have to make the most of our female advantage, even when real life intervenes.

The Structure of Sleep

Sleep has its own architecture, or structure, consisting of distinct stages. During the various stages of sleep, our muscles are in different states of relaxation, our nervous systems in different levels of arousal. And, of course, there are differences in brain activity and brain waves.

Sleep involves a number of brain functions, which integrate the chemical and electrical activity of our brain cells, the time of day, and the amount of sleep we've had and still need. Knowledge of those interactions aids your doctor in finding ways to help you if you have a sleep problem.

Over the years I have found that the explanation of sleep and wake is best kept simple. So we'll dispense with the usual brain wave charts. Instead, I want you to picture a child's seesaw with two balls on it. When the balls are of equal size and in similar places on either end of the seesaw, it remains in balance. If one of the balls is bigger or heavier, or a different distance from the center, the seesaw tips; the heavy end goes down. It is clear that the weight or placement of one ball affects the other. In other words, the balls interact in a general way, and aspects of each influence the other over your twenty-four-hour "day."

Your sleep and wake systems are much like those balls. In your mind's eye, label one ball "sleep" and the other "wake." Throughout this book I will talk of ways to keep these systems in balance or correct them if they are out of balance.

It's comforting to know that most of us are born with all the correct anatomy to sleep well and remain alert when we need to. When we're a few months old, our sleep systems should begin forming a stable structure and integrating with our wake systems to form a balance. This balance usually remains through childhood into puberty. Unfortunately, as we get older we seem to spend a great deal of effort unbalancing these systems. For instance, we push ourselves to do too much work, thinking we can sacrifice sleep. We switch our sleep schedule to accommodate

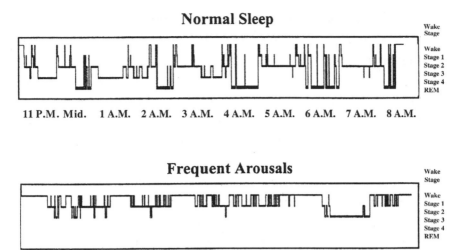

The difference between a good night's sleep and a restless night.

our daytime pressures. We eat and drink the wrong things, and we get sick. Many times the symptoms of other illnesses or the medications we take for them unbalance our sleep systems.

Your Sleep Cycles

In the sleep lab we can precisely chart the stages of sleep. We attach electrodes to the scalp, face, and legs to monitor brain waves and muscle tone, while other devices keep track of heart rate, breathing, body temperature, and even genital arousal and hormonal activity, if needed. Believe it or not, it's perfectly possible to get a good night's sleep in the lab, even with all those wires attached. We keep things quiet, dark, and peaceful, and we try to provide comfortable mattresses and pillows. Believe me, if you're very sleep-deprived, you'll fall asleep just about anywhere once the lights go out.

You may think that we slowly drift off to a deep sleep, have a few dreams, then slowly awaken. But that's not true. We cycle through different stages of sleep, some deeper than others, and not all of them are conducive to dreaming.

Our brains cycle into two main states of sleep, dream sleep or *REM (rapid eye movement sleep)* and *non-REM sleep (NREM)*. There are several depths to NREM sleep. They are called stages 1 through 4, to denote the "depth" of sleep, based on the brain's ability to awaken. Stages 3 and 4 are the deepest, when the brain's activity slows considerably; that's the slow-wave sleep I mentioned before, the deep, restorative sleep women are supposed to be getting more of.

When you're awake and alert, your brain is very active, producing electrical signals called *beta waves.* When you climb into bed and begin your descent into sleep, you enter a relaxed, half-awake state, a transitional, light-sleep stage *(stage 1 sleep).* This stage can last a few seconds to a few minutes. Brain activity slows down somewhat, producing mixed-frequency waves called *alpha* and *theta waves,* with slow, rolling eye movements. This is the stage during which you are "falling asleep." Some people actually experience a sensation of falling and may involuntarily jerk their muscles. (If your partner kicks you in bed when just falling asleep, it's probably during this stage.)

As you relax further, your breathing and heart rate slow down, and you enter the second stage of sleep, *stage 2.* Your brain activity also slows, producing brain waves at a mixed frequency of slower theta waves. Eventually you settle in, your breathing becomes regular, your heart rate stabilizes, and you enter stage 2 sleep. Many researchers consider this period, which may last ten to twenty minutes, the beginning of real sleep. During this period we stop moving around and muscle tension eases, and we are oblivious to outside stimulation (like street noise). During stage 2, theta waves mix with what we call sleep spindles, spindle-shaped beta waves that show little bursts of consolidating brain activity.

Then you move into *stage 3 sleep.* Theta waves mix with slower *delta waves,* which eventually dominate in *stage 4 sleep,* deep sleep. This is the sleep you need to feel rested, and it's very deep indeed. If a ringing telephone jolts you awake from deep sleep, you're apt to feel groggy and momentarily disoriented. You may remember being able to carry your young child from the car to bed shortly after she fell asleep and she never even stirred. That's because she was in deep sleep. It is very hard to awaken anyone of any age from this stage of sleep. Although we spend about 75 percent of the night in the different stages of NREM sleep, most of our deep sleep takes place in the first third of the night.

Finally, after about seventy to ninety minutes, REM sleep kicks in, and this dreaming state recurs every seventy to ninety minutes across the night (even though we may not remember our dreams). During dream sleep we have periods of what we call *tonic* (no muscle tone) and *phasic* activity. For instance, our eyes dart around as though they are watching our dreams unfold during the phasic periods. Fortunately, because of the lack of muscle tone, our bodies cannot move during this time. We are paralyzed. In fact, the only parts that do move are our eyes, diaphragms (breathing muscles), nasal membranes, and other erectile tissue, like the penis or clitoris (more about that in Chapter 6).

During REM sleep our heartbeats are irregular and our blood pressure can surge. We cannot control our temperatures either. Fortunately, REM sleep comes only in brief segments, sometimes a few minutes at a time, other times longer. Most REM sleep occurs in the last third of the night, or the early-morning hours (which is why your alarm clock often seems to awaken you in the middle of a dream).

After the first period of REM sleep, we awaken for a second or two, cycle back into stage 2, stage 3, and stage 4, then ascend for more dreaming. The length of each REM period increases through the night, so that the last one, in the early morning, may be twenty to forty minutes long. After this period of early-morning REM sleep, we typically wake up, feeling alert.

By now you're probably beginning to think that sleep can get complicated, but just remember that seesaw and the balls.

Although our brains continue to be active, our bodies are usually quiet during all of sleep. In the segments of NREM sleep, we appear to really rest.

Young children spend a lot of time, almost half the night, in deep sleep. We think that this is the most useful stage of sleep to build muscle, repair tissues, and clear cell damage that may have occurred during the day. As we age we get less and less recognizable deep sleep. Actually, I enjoy telling adult audiences that we are all over the hill: our best sleep occurs before we reach puberty. Sorry about that.

What Regulates Sleep?

Unless you're doing shift work, you most likely go to sleep when it's dark outside. This choice of sleep time is not a choice at all but a drive governed by our biological clock. This clock is located in a specific area of the brain behind the eyes (called the *suprachiasmatic nucleus*), which senses light and dark. When things are in balance, our biological clock regulates the time of our sleep as well as other body hormones. Some of those hormones (like melatonin and growth hormone) are closely linked to sleep; others are not. This drive to sleep at night is governed by our *circadian* (or twenty-four-hour) *rhythm*. Recent research has found that this rhythm has a genetic makeup as well. So "larks," those of us who rise early and function better in the daytime, and "owls," who come alive at night, may have inherited those tendencies.

Our circadian rhythm actually has two periods during the twenty-four-hour day in which we are most driven to sleep. The strongest sleep drive is between 2:00 and 4:00 A.M.; the second is between 1:00 and 3:00 P.M. You've probably experienced difficulty staying awake during those times. Many people incorrectly believe the afternoon dip of alertness is the result of eating a heavy lunch. Now you know better.

Conversely, the clock also promotes periods of wakefulness during our daytime hours. Strangely, this influence for wakefulness increases as the day goes on, so that our ability to sleep between 6:00 and 8:00 P.M. is very poor. These hours are labeled a forbidden zone for sleep!

It's also nice to know that we women hold on to our circadian rhythms longer as we age, so we may not be as likely as men to crawl into bed early at night only to awaken before dawn. However, our circadian rhythms can be disrupted by hormonal factors such as premenstrual syndrome or menopausal hot flashes (see Chapter 2).

Another sleep drive is called the *homeostatic drive.* That's simply the need for sleep that develops while we are awake. It's clearly related to how much wakefulness we've had. For instance, the longer we are awake, the stronger our need to sleep.

You can see how the circadian and homeostatic drives need to compete at the end of the day; one pushing wake, the other pushing sleep. As complex as the sleep and wake systems are (scientists are now exam-

Circadian and Homeostatic Drives for Sleep and Wake

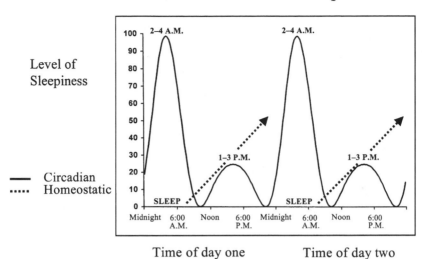

Level of
Sleepiness

— Circadian
..... Homeostatic

Time of day one   Time of day two

Your homeostatic drive to sleep (the upward arrows) builds the longer you stay awake . . . and is often at odds with your body clock, or circadian rhythm (the hills and valleys of natural alertness and sleepiness).

ining them on a molecular level), they are also simple when seen in this context. We clearly cause good and bad interactions on a daily basis, which can be scientifically documented on a cellular level.

For example, toxins and other chemicals build up when we are awake, and energy stores are depleted. One of the chemicals that build up and produce sleep is adenosine. Caffeine, which combats adenosine, has been shown in the fruit fly to reduce rest and enhance the wake-promoting influence of the circadian clock. We all know that a cup of coffee or tea can help recharge us during the day. But, because caffeine stays in the bloodstream, it also combats our sleep-making chemicals if taken too late (see page 32).

On average, for optimal functioning, most of us need between seven and nine hours of sleep a night. Most of us get less. Some of us need even more, as much as ten hours. Every time we cut our sleep short, even by a few minutes, that period of sleep loss accumulates. If we lose sleep every night, eventually the sleep loss overcomes us. We find ourselves

What About Jet Lag?

One of the most common disrupters of circadian rhythm is jet lag. This occurs when we cross several time zones, going either east or west (it doesn't happen when we fly north or south). Eastward flights can shorten your day by several hours, depending on how many time zones you cross; westward flights lengthen the day. Even though you're in a new time zone, your sleep and wake patterns remain set to your *home* zone. The result: sleep fragmentation, frequent awakenings, poor-quality, non-restorative sleep, and daytime sleepiness. Jet lag can even lead to depression, muscle aches, headaches, and stomach upsets.

You can avoid jet lag if you time your flights right and give yourself enough time to adjust to the new time zone, especially to light and dark cues. I advise people to follow the sun. When you take a night flight, avoid alcohol and snooze on the plane (take a sleep aid, preferably by prescription). The next day, get out in the sunlight as soon as possible. If you hop on a morning flight, go to bed at your normal time (even if the new time zone puts you a couple of hours later) to stay in sync with your natural sleep patterns. Recent studies show that taking melatonin (see page 68) does *not* help prevent jet lag.

falling asleep unexpectedly. We may also feel and act irritable beforehand. Finding out your personal sleep need is very important, even if you cannot always get the sleep you need. At least you'll know when you're in jeopardy of being cranky and having a sleep attack. Sleep attacks can come when you least expect them, and even though they may be short (under twenty seconds), they can cause lots of damage if they occur while you are doing a crucial job like driving. When the two sleep drives (circadian and homeostatic) combine, for instance at 4:00 A.M. after twenty hours of wakefulness, it is almost impossible to stay awake. Not surprisingly, that's the peak time for automobile accidents. Sleepy people do not make safe drivers. Sleepy mothers do not make good carpoolers. People who drink and drive, especially when they're sleepy, are at even more risk because alcohol enhances sleep loss.

One Australian study compared hours of sleep loss to levels of blood alcohol and found that seventeen hours of wakefulness was equivalent to having a blood alcohol level of 0.05 percent—enough in some states to be considered legally drunk. If folks were up for twenty-four hours straight, their functioning was equal to those with a blood alcohol level of 0.1 percent—definitely drunk! Even worse, researchers at Henry Ford Hospital note that the combination of alcohol and sleep loss makes each one that much worse.

To test how much sleep you need, try sleeping as long as you can for several days during a vacation and see how well you can stay awake in some quiet, boring situation. If you are falling asleep, chances are your homeostatic drive is telling you that you are getting too little sleep. Check out page 15 for a simple test to see if you're too sleepy.

Now there are women who function quite well on six hours of sleep. But "function well" is the operative phrase here. If you're able to work, stay up well past midnight, wake with no trouble at 6:30 A.M., and stay alert, then whatever amount of sleep you're getting is probably adequate for you. But if you find yourself drowsy after lunch, sleepy during your commute, or dozing in front of the TV after dinner, you're probably sleep-deprived. Ditto if you fall asleep the minute your head hits the pillow (or don't even remember climbing into bed!). This is a great clue. We actually feel that taking about fifteen minutes to fall asleep is "normal," and that a problem doesn't exist until people consistently take more than twenty minutes to fall asleep.

The important thing is to consider why you are sleep-deprived. Maybe you don't allow yourself enough time to sleep, or perhaps the sleep you get is disrupted in some way. Incidentally, some self-described short sleepers forget to mention that they take restorative short naps during the day.

Why We Need Sleep

Why do our bodies *need* to sleep? Strangely, sleep researchers still can't answer that question. There are many theories. Some scientists think we sleep to repair our cells or rest the building blocks of our bodies and minds. That is a tempting idea when we think of how much small children need to sleep and how quickly they grow.

Metabolic activity and body temperature are both reduced while we sleep, conserving energy and providing a chance for tissues to grow and repair. Blood supply to our muscles increases during deep sleep, allowing the body to recover from the physical stresses of the day. In fact, deep sleep increases the night after you've had a day of vigorous exercise (probably because of increased brain temperature, a side effect of exercise. See page 26).

Many researchers agree that one role of dream sleep is to stimulate the brain with volleys of electrical activity. Recent studies suggest that sleep may play a vital role in learning and memory processing. Some experts believe that we need dream sleep to help sort out and store memories. REM sleep and dreams also appear to be crucial for mental performance. (I'll talk more about dreams—and how to use them—in Chapter 5.)

A new study from Harvard Medical School found for the first time that getting a good night's sleep is key to forming certain kinds of memories. The study found that when students didn't get at least six to eight hours of sleep, newly acquired information didn't get properly encoded into the brain's "memory circuits." And it was not just the amount of sleep: the students needed both deep, slow-wave sleep *and* REM sleep to properly encode memory and enhance learning.

Conversely, the brain may be adversely affected by sleep deprivation because certain patterns of electrical and chemical activity that normally occur during sleep get interrupted. In fact, a study from the University of California at San Diego found that the ability of the brain to cope with cognitive tasks is altered after sleep deprivation, lessening the ability to perform cognitive tasks. The study of thirteen students showed that although the brain compensates by activating different areas to help with the task at hand, certain areas simply weren't up to the task, such as those involved in arithmetic problems. The sleepy students made more mistakes and left out more answers.

There's research to suggest that sleep is critically linked to the immune system, and that a lack of sleep may make us more vulnerable to colds and other bugs. We all know how much more sleep we seem to need when we are sick and feverish. Fever induces sleep. We used to think that was simply the body healing itself. We now know that factors

How Sleepy Are You?

This simple questionnaire can help you determine whether you're suffering from excessive daytime sleepiness. Just rate how likely you would be to doze off in any of the following situations. Your answers are rated using the Epworth Sleepiness Scale. The scale ranges from 0 to 3, with 0 meaning you'd never doze off or fall asleep in a given situation and 3 meaning there's a good chance you'd nod off. To get your score, add up the numbers you put after each situation. This scale should not be used to make a diagnosis. It's simply a tool to help you identify how sleepy you are during the day, which is a symptom of many sleep disorders.

Choose the most appropriate number for each situation:
0=Would never doze
1=Slight chance of dozing
2=Moderate chance of dozing
3=High chance of dozing

Situation	Chance of Dozing
Sitting and reading	_____
Watching television	_____
Sitting inactive in a public place (e.g., a theater or meeting)	_____
As a passenger in a car for an hour without a break	_____
Lying down to rest in the afternoon	_____
Sitting and talking to someone	_____
Sitting quietly after lunch (when you've had no alcohol)	_____
In a car, when stopped for traffic	_____
YOUR SCORE	_____

A score of less than 8 means that you're not suffering from excessive daytime sleepiness. A score of 10 or more means you may need to think more about your sleep. If your score is 15 or more, please share this information with your physician, describing all your sleep-related symptoms.

Remember, true excessive daytime sleepiness is almost always caused by an underlying medical condition that usually can be easily diagnosed and effectively treated.

Source: Murray W. Johns, M.D., director of the Sleep Center at Epworth Hospital, Melbourne, Australia. Reproduced with permission of the author.

in the blood called cytokines (specifically interleukin-6, or IL-6) may be to blame. These are modulators of the immune system. IL-6 is an inflammatory cytokine that causes the symptoms of sleepiness and may have detrimental effects on the cardiovascular system and bones.

Measures of IL-6 decline during sleep and are elevated on the day after sleep deprivation. In fact, it may be the elevation that is responsible for our sleepy feeling the following day. The total amount of IL-6 does not change over the twenty-four-hour period, just the rhythm of its secretion. So, along with an increase of IL-6 and the symptoms of sleepiness in the day, the following night's sleep may be deeper because IL-6 secretion is lower. Good sleep may lessen the wear and tear from substances like IL-6.

Stress is also a mediator of our immune system, possibly through sleep! When we are stressed, we sleep poorly, and we also seem more prone to illnesses. A recent study measured stress (intrusive/avoidance thoughts) in humans and noted that as stress increased, time spent awake during the sleep period increased, and levels of "natural killer cells," which protect us from germs, went down. Poor sleep following natural disasters and other incidents of stress has been linked with a decrease in natural killer cells.

Chronic sleep loss may also hasten some aspects of aging. Recent studies under the direction of Dr. Eve Van Cauter at the University of Chicago found that lack of sleep can alter hormone levels and affect the body's ability to burn carbohydrates. One study found that a single week of sleep deprivation hindered glucose metabolism and slowed the body's ability to secrete the hormone insulin (which regulates blood sugar). These effects could conceivably speed the onset (or increase the severity of) age-related, type 2 diabetes. In addition, sleep-deprived people had higher nighttime levels of the stress hormone cortisol (which also regulates blood sugar) and lower levels of thyroid-stimulating hormone, which affects metabolism. The good news is that once the subjects got more sleep, their hormone levels returned to normal. But if you're chronically sleep-deprived, your body may adapt and the changes could become irreversible. Authors of this study likened sleep deprivation to stress, which can have effects on the brain that cause memory loss. We also know that stress leads to poor sleep and, consequently, poor immunity or health. Regardless of why sleep is disturbed, this relationship may occur.

Additionally, studies have shown that disrupting the sleep of healthy young people caused significant body pain. One recent study suggests disruptions in slow-wave sleep may lower the pain threshold for women suffering musculoskeletal disorders such as arthritis and fibromyalgia (and may even play a role in that disorder). Sleep loss can also cause personal disaster. Take a look at your local newspaper and see how many times you read of a single-occupant car accident in the wee hours of the morning, where the cause is unknown. The paper typically reads: "The weather and roadway were fine. It is still unknown why the car drove off the road and hit the tree (or something else)." The likelihood is that the driver fell asleep, however briefly, and missed a turn or hit a bridge.

Whatever the reasons we sleep, we know that we simply cannot do without sleep. Just like food and water, sleep is an essential part of our lives. We certainly would not expect to go an entire day in the heat without water. Why should we expect that we could go without sleep just because we're busy? We show signs of sleep deprivation just as we show signs of hunger. We know we get cranky and forgetful when we shortcut our sleep. We may not realize how dramatically our reaction times and decision-making abilities slow. We won't be able to stay awake, even if we try to, when sleep loss is severe enough.

An important fact to remember is that sleep occurs in boring or warm, cozy situations *because* we are sleep-deprived. It is not true that boring situations cause sleepiness.

Common Sleep Disrupters

As I mentioned, our sleep is very often disrupted by hormonal factors unique to women. But other things that interfere with a good night's sleep also affect women more often than men.

For one thing, we suffer disproportionately from pain, including arthritis, headaches, and pain syndromes such as fibromyalgia.

What we eat—and don't eat—can also affect sleep. For example, a deficiency in calcium, magnesium, or iron (and many younger women are iron-deficient without knowing it) might lead to wakefulness. Recent research has linked iron deficiency to restless legs syndrome (see page 145). Calcium and magnesium appear to have a sedative effect; a great time to take calcium supplements is in the evening. Studies show most women are getting only half the calcium they need, which may not only weaken our bones but also disrupt our sleep. Not to mention that calcium may help reduce some symptoms of premenstrual syndrome, which also keeps some women awake nights. (For more about calcium and magnesium, see pages 53–54.)

Far too many of us are chronic dieters. If you're eating too little, hunger can make you restless and prevent a good night's sleep. A low-carbohydrate diet may also hamper your sleep, because carbohydrates help send the sleep-inducing amino acid tryptophan to the brain.

We've all succumbed to an attack of the munchies in the evening. But overeating (especially too close to bedtime) can lead to indigestion and a restless night, whereas a proper pre-bedtime snack can help ensure a good night's sleep (see page 40). By the way, lack of sleep may also lead us to eat too much. Some studies have reported that people who are sleep-deprived have an increased appetite. They may not only eat more but eat more of the wrong kinds of foods as a reflex to increase brain glucose to try to stay awake. The result: weight gain.

Many women are using alcohol as a sleep aid, not knowing it can actually interfere with sleep. A drink or two may relax you and make you feel sleepy, but after you get into bed and the alcohol is processed by your body, it will wake you (see pages 34–37). Alcohol is also a diuretic; it will make you get up to empty your bladder during the night.

Another sleep robber is smoking. A study at the University of Kansas found that cigarette smokers were more likely to experience poor sleep, daytime sleepiness, and minor accidents, and to consume more caffeine. Nicotine is a stimulant and raises heart rate and blood pressure. Not to mention that women smokers are more prone to lung cancer than men.

I once had a patient who complained of chronic insomnia. We tried all the sleep hygiene techniques, to no avail. She had reported a moder-

---

Top Ten Sleep Busters

- Stress or anxiety
- Illness
- Noise
- Light
- Poor schedule

- Caffeine
- Alcohol
- Stimulant medications
- Depression or anger
- Fear or poor security

---

ate smoking habit but neglected to tell us that she smoked all her cigarettes during the night. She would awaken almost every hour and have a cigarette to "relax" her back to sleep. Needless to say, she was not pleased at the thought of discontinuing her habit, but ultimately that was the only way she could get a good night's sleep.

Want to sleep better? Stop smoking.

Women suffer from major depression twice as often as men, and sleeping too much (or too little) is one of the classic signs of major depression, as is having trouble falling asleep. Insomnia is a common symptom of dysthymia (a mild but chronic form of depression). Low self-esteem and chronic fatigue can also be signs of this form of depression. When the days get short and the nights long, some people suffer from seasonal affective disorder (SAD), which not only brings about depression and irritability but also causes people to sleep more and sometimes feel sleepy during the day.

The other symptoms of major depression include losing interest in normally pleasurable activities and feeling sad, hopeless, helpless, and worthless. You may also feel fatigued or slowed down, experience appetite changes, weight loss or weight gain, headaches, stomachaches, back pain, or pains in muscles or joints that do not seem to respond to treatment. If you have thoughts of suicide, please get help immediately. Depression can be treated. You do not have to feel this way!

The same goes for anxiety. Anxiety disorders are the most common mental health problem affecting Americans and are twice as common in women. Signs of anxiety disorders include excessive worry that interferes with daily activities and keeps you awake nights (sometimes accompanied by rapid or pounding heartbeats). Generalized anxiety disorder may cause stress during the day and interfere with sleep.

Depression and anxiety can take you by surprise at any time, but particularly after having a baby or during the years before menopause, when your hormones are fluctuating greatly.

You'll need to choose antidepressants carefully, since some can interfere with sleep (anxiety medications often have a mild sedating effect). Remember, the brain uses the same chemicals to regulate sleep as it does to regulate mood. If there is an imbalance in mood, or an overabundance of anxiety, chances are that sleep systems will be out of balance, too. Remember the seesaw and balls? Anxiety will "puff up" the wake ball, so sleep cannot get a chance to take over.

If you think you may be depressed (or suffer from anxiety), don't hesitate to tell your doctor; these problems are usually very treatable. And treatment will vastly improve your sleep! Seasonal affective disorder is treated with both antidepressants and light therapy (see Chapter 4).

Learning the Four Rs of Sleep

To get a better night's sleep, you need to strengthen your natural female sleep systems, so you can get that extra slow-wave sleep women are supposed to have.

You can take some basic steps to help accomplish this. Some sleep specialists call them sleep hygiene. My colleague Dr. Joan Shaver of the University of Illinois at Chicago has dubbed these steps the Four Rs of Sleep:

• **Regularize** your sleep-wake patterns. Get up at the same time daily. Avoid naps, unless they are regular. Try to sleep the same amount each night. Find the perfect amount of sleep time for you and stick with it.

• **Ritualize** cues for good sleep. Use the bedroom only for sleep and sex. Keep the environment quiet, dark, cool, and safe for sleeping. Go to bed only when you're sleepy.

• **Relax.** Find ways to reduce stress and control tension. Learn some relaxation techniques. Try yoga or biofeedback. Start a worry book (see page 27).

• **Resist** behaviors that interfere with sleep: keep away from alcohol, tobacco, and caffeine. Avoid strenuous exercise within three hours of bedtime. And don't eat heavy meals before bed.

Regularize

Of Dr. Shaver's Four Rs, regularizing sleep-wake patterns is perhaps the most important.

Remember those two balls and the seesaw? One ball is sleep, one is wake. When we keep regular hours, we help our biological clock stay on rhythm. It's easiest to keep a regular wake time, because we can usually force ourselves awake. Forcing ourselves to fall asleep is impossible.

We also want to keep regular daytime activities; regular mealtimes, regular exercise patterns, and regular exposure to daylight, so that our biological clocks know night from day, and consequently sleep from wake.

Many of us spend our days in a work environment lit by fluorescent light, then go home to a house that's lit until midnight or after. So our biological propensity to sleep in the dark may be wiped out; the body doesn't see drastic changes anymore between day and night, light and dark. And, certainly as we get older, we need to increase that difference to give ourselves good cues for sleep as our sleep patterns shift.

Similarly, people work all day, then go home and work some more, or they watch television or surf the Internet. You may be functioning in work-alert mode for eighteen to twenty hours out of twenty-four. For many of us, the body doesn't get a chance to switch from active day to relaxed night, and that's dangerous. We wind up not sleeping terribly well and can't figure out why. So give yourself some time in the evening to wind down and prepare your body for sleep.

Ritualize

What do I mean by "ritualizing cues" for sleep? Darkness is a cue for sleep to our biological clock. Have shades or curtains that will close out the daylight, particularly if you're in a well-lit city area or work the night shift. Light therapy can also help a disrupted sleep-wake cycle (see page 161).

Use earplugs or sound-muffling gadgets to filter out sounds from other household members or street noise. Many people swear that "white noise," be it the hum of an air conditioner or one of those machines that make sounds like waves lapping the shore, helps them sleep. That's a personal preference. If it helps you, fine. However, I draw the line at playing the radio softly. We know that people can adjust to their environment (think of those folks who live near airports), but research shows that sound does disturb the brain during sleep, even though we may not recognize it. (The converse is leaving your noisy neighborhood for a quiet country inn and not being able to sleep.) And, remember, even on all-music radio stations, the pitch and tempo of the music change, announcers announce. The basic idea is to have quiet.

A sensible, comforting mattress (soft or firm) helps you sleep. I'm often asked about mattress types. Really, that's a choice best left to each sleeper. You should do a lot of testing before you buy, and pick what feels right to you.

I advise a slightly cool room temperature for sleep, since it's easier to get warm than it is to cool off. Ideally, we'd all be better off (sleep-wise, that is) with a private sleep space rather than sharing space with a roommate or partner who's noisy or keeps separate hours, or a bedmate who snores, makes noises, or thrashes and disrupts our sleep.

Of course, we make accommodations for spouses, for children, and for other life events. But, in essence, if we are having trouble sleeping, we need to set a quiet, serene, cocoonlike area in which we can let sleep happen.

Reserving the bedroom for sleep and sex seems like a pretty obvious idea, but many people overlook it. Stress does not make a good bedfellow. That means you don't tackle your taxes in the bedroom, or continue an argument in bed. If sex at bedtime isn't satisfying or relaxing, pick an alternate time when you can be less stressed. You don't want to increase your stress level in any way just before trying to sleep.

Because surveys indicate that not feeling safe can interfere with sleep, you might also want to ritualize "security checks" if this is an issue for you. Before you retire, be sure doors and windows are closed and locked, alarm systems on. If you make this routine, you won't wake in the middle of the night wondering whether you left that window open.

Another way to strengthen your sleep system is to ban glow-in-the-dark bedroom clocks. They're handy devices, but they can also sabotage your sleep. If you need an alarm to wake up, set your alarm, then turn the clock away or cover it, so you can't check on it. It should be comforting to know that we all awaken during the night—actually after every REM period—four to five times a night. This is a perfectly normal phenomenon. Most of us, who are not particularly anxious, don't recognize it as being awake. We unconsciously reposition ourselves, roll over, and go back to sleep. But if you are aware of these brief awakenings, because your anxiety is a little greater, you've had a stressful day, or you have a problem on your mind, you may be more tuned in to the fact that you have awakened. One look at the bedroom clock reinforces that awake feeling. This begins a negative cycle. If it's early in the night, you say, "Oh no, I'm starting to wake up already." If it's late you say, "Oh my God, it's almost morning and I've gotten very little sleep." Some people swear they wake up during the night at the same time every night when they're having a bout of insomnia. How do they know? Take one guess. They have unconsciously taught themselves to awaken at a specific time by watching the clock!

Time should have no importance at night. The lesson here is to understand that you should be asleep when it's dark out and you're in your bed. It shouldn't matter what time it is; whether you have one hour or six hours to go should not be a concern. You know that your alarm is set; if you don't look at the clock, you'll fall back asleep more easily. Hiding the clock may not be effective the first night or the second, but it will certainly help you by the end of the week, and you'll find that it's a miraculous cure for those midnight or middle-of-the-night awakenings.

Many of my colleagues tell patients that if they can't fall asleep they should get out of bed after ten minutes and do some quiet activity. But too many women are driven today by "should dos" and may jump to get up because they want to finish office work they've brought home, a hem they were repairing, or some household chore. So I usually tell women to stay in bed unless they're really agitated. To put yourself in a relaxed state for sleep, get comfortable in bed, try to clear your mind. Concentrate on a sound or sensation (such as breathing) to ward off competing signals. Think of a pleasant spot (like the beach) and imagine yourself there.

If you find that you're tossing and turning for more than twenty or thirty minutes, and getting anxious about falling asleep (your heart is racing and your breathing is faster), get up! There's no point in staying in bed under those circumstances.

Find something relaxing to do, preferably in a darkened, quiet environment. I would *not* suggest television, since we may tune in to a show that's too stimulating, and the light from the television can also be stimulating to our biological clock! Sometimes sitting by a window or sitting with a very dim light trying to read, stretch, knit, or do some relaxation exercises will be very helpful. When you begin to feel sleepy again, go back to bed.

Many women tell me that they need to get up to go to the bathroom in the middle of the night. Research has shown that we don't have to urinate that often. If you get up to pee in the night, chances are not much comes out. It's very typical for folks during a normal awakening to say, "Oh, I must have woken up because I have to go to the bathroom." So they get up and go into the bathroom, perhaps turning on a light, again reinforcing awakening, just to piddle. If you find that this is an issue, say repeatedly to yourself, "I don't have to pee," and return to sleep. Of course, this doesn't take into account physical problems such as overactive bladder or incontinence, which affect women more often than men (see pages 110–11), or apnea, which alters the body's excretion of urine.

Exercise is another useful tool for regularizing sleep. It can help burn off stress as well as fat (both of which, by the way, can contribute to women's risk of heart disease). However, while there are a number of benefits to improved conditioning (you'll build muscle, burn body fat, help keep bones strong), there's no data to suggest that exercise will *prevent* sleepiness. What it helps to do is raise body and brain temperatures. Slow-wave sleep also acts to lower brain temperature. So the higher the temperature, the deeper the sleep. (Remember how sleepy you are with a fever?) By the way, this may have something to do with why men fall asleep so quickly after sexual activity (see page 184).

Can You "Catch Up" on Lost Sleep?

Too many of us grab whatever sleep we can during the week and try to catch up by sleeping in on the weekends. But maintaining the same amount of sleep time each night also helps strengthen your sleep system. If you sleep for eight or nine hours on the weekend to make up sleep loss during the week, you may disrupt your sleep on Sunday night. Many cases of insomnia start just this way. Such a pattern also begins a cycle of work-week sleep deprivation. It takes a week to "repay" a sleep debt and reach your optimal number of sleep hours. So a good time to add on extra sleep is on vacation.

Of course, not all of us have the option of sleeping longer. So here are steps you can take when there literally aren't enough hours in the day or night.

• Remain consistent. Try to get the same amount of sleep each night (even if it's shorter). Try adding fifteen minutes each night when you can. Get out of bed at the same time each day. Although it's okay to sleep an extra hour or so, you may find your body waking you up anyway.

• Take naps when you can. They are great refreshers. Try taking twenty-minute naps on a consistent basis, even one in the morning and one in the afternoon (if your schedule allows). Coffee-break time can begin with a short nap and end with a stimulating cup of java. This will refresh you for a couple of hours.

• Light is a good pick-me-up. Try to get outdoors for part of the day. You can still use sunscreen to protect your skin. What counts here is light coming through your eyes to the brain center that controls your twenty-four-hour biological clock. If you're tired, sunlight helps to reinforce the body's sense of daytime/wake time.

• Make sleep a priority. When work requires longer hours or you're traveling, make sure to get back to your schedule as soon as you can. If need be, give up nonessential activities, but get your sleep.

But be careful what time you choose to exercise. Exercise is initially stimulating. So for some people vigorous exercise right before bed can limit sleep and prolong its onset. However, recent studies show that for other people exercise within an hour or two of bed has no effect or may even promote sleep. Still, for someone with insomnia, the best time for exercise is late afternoon or early evening. The general recommendation is to exercise at least three hours before bedtime. But if evening is the only time you can exercise, go to it. It's better than being inactive. Yoga and stretching are wonderful nighttime exercises, since they relax you and could improve your ability to fall asleep.

Speaking of raising your body temperature, taking a hot bath an hour or so before bedtime can also set you up nicely for sleep. I'm talking water that's at least 100 degrees Fahrenheit, and a soak of more than thirty minutes. After your body temperature is raised, it will fall once you lie down in a cool room. And that will send you off to sleep more quickly and promote more deep sleep. (A note of caution: If you have high blood pressure or a heart condition, or are prone to dizziness, consult your doctor before you try very hot baths.)

Relax

Along with reinforcing our sleep mechanisms, we also need to reduce the amount of stress, anxiety, and worry that we carry around. Because it's sure to affect our sleep. A 1999 Roper survey found that women feel more stressed than men (especially full-time working mothers with children under age thirteen). Women also report worrying more than men. That's because of our multiple roles as wives, mothers, workers, and caretakers.

One way to reduce your worry level is to organize a time during the day when you can "worry well." Pick a time and place for your daily worry, then sit for a regimented half hour every day in this quiet, private area (yes, even a bathroom), and worry well.

To worry well, you'll also need a "worry book." My colleague Dr. Peter Hauri of the Mayo Clinic came up with the idea of writing down worries to help sleep (see his book *No More Sleepless Nights,* by Peter Hauri, M.D., and Shirley Linde, Ph.D., John Wiley and Sons, 1996). Dr. Hauri used index cards, but I recommend a child's school notebook. On the left-hand side of the page list the issues that have been running through your head, and on the right-hand side list some forward motion on those worries.

For example, a left-side entry might read: "Mary was really strange today at work. She snapped at me. What did I do? What was she really saying? Maybe she overheard that comment I made about her weight. I didn't mean to say it, it just popped out. She'll never forgive me." On the right side of the page you might write: "I will ask Mary if everything is okay. I will tell her how upset I was that she snapped at me and ask if I upset her in some way. If she mentions the remark, I'll apologize and tell her that I value her friendship. Everyone says something stupid once in a while."

Maybe you've been worried about money. On the left-hand side you might write: "Money, money, money. There's just never enough. We have six bills due at the end of the week, and how can I pay for the kids' braces and the car repairs? And our taxes are due next month! I just never catch up!" Then, on the right side you might write: "I will balance my checkbook tomorrow and go over all our accounts. I know I can find some ways to economize. I'll put off buying that new outfit I wanted. I'll use the money I put aside for clothes for the car repairs. I'll file a tax extension, call an accountant, and see if there are some ways to reduce the tax bill."

Using the worry book, you not only list your worries but jot down some potential solutions to the problems. You accomplish several things by doing this. First, all of those worries that run through your head at night may, in fact, be able to be condensed to a very few issues during waking daytime hours. It may be very hard to find the issues that bothered you during the night. You'll begin to understand that you may have anxiety patterns. There may be a work issue, there may be a family issue, but in black and white and during the day it may not be quite so large as it feels in the dark when you can't sleep, and it may be fairly easily resolved. Feeling that you can find solutions to problems and that they are not going to get the better of you is empowering and comforting. And you needn't rush. It can take days or weeks to resolve the problems that may appear on the left-hand side of the page. This is a way to worry productively.

Stress: What's Going On?

I don't have to tell you that stress is a major sleep buster.

What's happening to our bodies when we're under stress? Experts generally define *stress* as feeling emotionally or physically threatened and feeling unable to do anything about it. *Burnout* is just another word for when stress piles up and we feel unable to cope.

When we're threatened, a primitive fight or flight response is triggered in our bodies. It sends a signal to the brain that in turn activates the sympathetic nervous system to produce stress hormones such as adrenaline and noradrenaline. These hormones increase heart rate, blood pressure, and breathing to send more blood and oxygen to the parts of the body that need it, such as muscles in the arms and legs, so we can flee the danger. Sugar and fats are released into the blood for quick energy. Once we're out of danger, the nervous system produces hormones like acetylcholine to counteract these effects, and we calm down.

Back in prehistoric days, the fight or flight response helped a human to escape a charging saber-toothed tiger. In the twenty-first century, however, this same response may be triggered by an angry boss or spouse, a screaming baby, too much work to do, or even a traffic jam that makes us late. Our own anger also produces this physiologic response.

If stress becomes chronic, the body may produce abnormal levels of stress hormones. Recent research indicates that women may have a heightened biological response to stress, producing more of certain stress hormones than men do. And stress hormones keep us awake. Stress leads to chronic anxiety, another sleep buster.

You may not always recognize symptoms of stress. Under extreme stress, your heart may pound, you may breathe hard and become flushed from the extra blood supply. But chronic stress can also trigger headaches, stomachaches, tight, achy muscles (especially in the back and shoulders), sweaty palms, all in addition to sleep difficulties. Your hands may tremble, you may get diarrhea or constipation, or break out in a rash or hives. You may feel dizzy or light-headed or have heartburn. Recent studies find that people under stress are even more likely to catch frequent colds; stress lowers the body's immune responses.

Emotional symptoms include nervousness, anxiety, crying, or feeling on edge, angry, and under pressure. You may also feel drained, powerless, lonely, self-doubting, or unhappy. Just about everything upsets you, you want to escape, and you may even have suicidal thoughts.

There are behavioral symptoms of chronic stress as well, things we do without thinking, such as eating compulsively, teeth grinding or biting nails, chain-smoking or drinking to excess. Some people continually show up late for work or go on shopping sprees. Others just anesthetize themselves with television.

Stress can cloud our thinking, sap our creativity, make us forgetful, indecisive, and unable to get things done. Chronic stress sends our sense of humor out the window.

When symptoms such as these occur together and repeatedly, they may be warning signs that the second silent killer—stress—is at work.

If you do begin to worry at night, you need to tell yourself: "I am not going there, I have done my worrying today, I'll do it tomorrow. I've forgotten nothing, tomorrow I will go back where I left it and I'll be fine. I should not be worrying now, and I won't."

Again, this is all assuming that there is no psychiatric disorder, such as depression or anxiety, driving those thoughts that prevent sleep. If you suspect you might have one of these disorders, please see a mental health professional without delay.

Some people may find that getting organized for the next day helps clear their heads of anxieties and worries: Did the kids pack their homework? Where's that report I need for my meeting? I'm going to be late tomorrow night, what shall I defrost for dinner? Some people find that taking care of small but key tasks, like setting out clothing, packing the kids' backpacks, writing notes to themselves and their partners, is a way to relieve the mind of burdens that can interfere with sleep. I definitely recommend this for busy people. It's also useful for kids and prevents those before-school hassles that can ruin a day before it begins.

Stress Busters for Women

Anything that relaxes the mind will help relax the body. But some relaxation techniques help more than others.

According to work by Dr. Herbert Benson, director of the Mind-Body Institute and chief of Behavioral Medicine at Beth Israel Deaconess Medical Center in Boston, relaxation exercises, yoga, and meditation all counterbalance the fight or flight reaction to stress by eliciting a "relaxation response" from the body. This response lowers heart rate and blood pressure, and slows breathing, calming you down so you can think more clearly.

How do you do this? Each technique uses a mental focusing device, such as repeating a word, sound, image, or physical activity. That way you can shake off thoughts that distract or worry you.

Biofeedback is used as a treatment for insomnia, since it helps you learn to relax. As you become conscious of normally *un*conscious body functions, such as muscle tension or breathing (the *bio* part), and using sounds or visual cues from electronic devices (the *feedback),* you can actually learn how to change or control those physiologic activities.

The biofeedback technique used most often to treat insomnia, called electromyography, or EMG biofeedback, measures muscle tension. In this technique electrodes leading to a monitor are attached to a specific muscle group or area of the body (which may be related to muscle tension or pain that keeps you awake). You'll be asked to consciously relax those muscles. Depending on the device, you'll get beeps or a tone signal, plus some sort of visual readout that changes along with the activity detected by the electrode as you perform the relaxation exercises. Once you've mastered the technique, you'll be able to produce that result without the machine.

You can do the same muscle relaxation exercises without any machine. To perform progressive muscle relaxation, close your eyes and with each breath imagine the tension draining away from your head muscles, your neck, and so on. This technique is most effective if you are lying down in a quiet place. You might also start from the toes up, first tightening each muscle group, then relaxing it.

Yoga, a form of gentle stretching exercise, is also relaxing. It relieves muscle stress and, we hope, the pain that interferes with sleep (unless you're new to yoga and very gung-ho and strain a muscle). Yoga not only relaxes and tones your muscles but has the potential to rest your mind as you "zone" into another space.

Meditation is somewhat different because of the lack of muscle movement. Meditation doesn't have to involve anything more exotic than sitting or lying comfortably in a relatively quiet place and letting your mind clear as you try to focus on breathing or muscle relaxation. You can repeat a word or phrase (called a *mantra*) to distract you from stressful thoughts or events. (Common mantras are *one, peace,* or *om.* You've probably done this before without realizing it; think of saying prayers in a quiet, darkened place). Some experts believe people who meditate actually fall into stage 1 sleep. A good meditation goes on for twenty to forty minutes, the equivalent of a nice, short nap! If while you focus on your breath or mantra, thoughts intrude, simply ignore them and return to your focus. Start with five minutes of meditation and work your way up.

Visualization can also help relax and ease you off to sleep. Try this exercise: Close your eyes and, using all of your senses, re-create in your mind a place where you've spent happy, relaxing times (perhaps the beach or a lake, the woods, a cabin in winter). Take the time to recall all the colors of your special place, how your body felt being there (the warmth of the sun on your skin, for example), even the smells and sounds. Picture all the details of your special place, then mentally take yourself there. When you get distracted, gently bring yourself back to the scene by focusing on the details.

Aromatherapy is another way to transport yourself to another place and relax. Essential oils of lavender, chamomile, and tangerine leaf are among those said to induce relaxation. Oils can also be found in sprays and lotions. Dab a drop of lavender oil on your pillowcase. If you take hot baths, try one of these scents in bath oil. Or make an aromatherapy sleep potion: Combine 3 drops lemon-balm oil, 3 drops lavender oil, and 1 drop rose oil in a small pot, simmer, and breathe in to relieve insomnia and stress. Do not use undiluted essential oils on your skin; they can cause allergic reactions. Before using any bath oil, do a "patch" test with a tiny drop on your skin. If the skin turns red and itchy, avoid that oil.

This is only a small sample of the ways you can help yourself relax before sleep. There are also a variety of tapes and self-help books available. So experiment. I've listed some resources in Appendix II.

Resist Caffeine

When trying to calm your wake system, resist stimulating foods and drugs. Number-one rule: Limit caffeine. If you are having difficulty falling asleep at night, I advise avoiding any caffeinated food or beverage from the afternoon on. It takes between fifteen and thirty minutes for the amount of caffeine in a cup of coffee (80 to 115 milligrams, depending on how it's made) to start acting on the brain, and around an hour to reach peak levels in the blood. Then caffeine is slowly broken down by the liver. It takes three to seven hours to completely rid your system of caffeine (depending on how old you are and how tolerant you are of caffeine). So that 3:00 P.M. cup of coffee may still be affecting you at bedtime.

Of course, not everyone is affected by caffeine. But if you get a big pick-me-up from a cup of coffee, switch to decaf in the afternoon. The same goes for tea. By the way, lattes and cappuccinos are made with the same one ounce of espresso diluted with milk. The quantity of caffeine stays the same, it's just in a bigger cup. Speaking of cups, take a look at your favorite coffee mug. Chances are that a big mug is the equivalent of two cups of coffee!

Limit colas and other soft drinks, some of which pack an even bigger wallop of caffeine, and caffeinated waters (like Java Water), which contain almost as much caffeine as coffee. Chocolate, coffee, and chocolate or coffee ice cream and yogurt all contain caffeine. So read labels carefully.

I would also check any medications you're taking to see if they contain caffeine or other products that tend to be stimulating. For example, Excedrin Migraine, Dexatrim, and the prescription headache medicines Fiorinal (butalbital, aspirin, and caffeine) and Fioricet (butalbital, acetaminophen, and caffeine) all have caffeine as an active ingredient. (See box on page 35). Caffeine can help relieve headaches, but if you take these pills at night, they can keep you awake. Methysergide, a medication that aborts headaches, can also cause sleeplessness.

Other medications that can hamper sleep include certain antidepressants, especially monoamine oxidase inhibitors (MAOIs), bronchodilating drugs, such as those used for asthma, steroids, some

How Much Caffeine in My Latte?

Food	Serving Size	Milligrams of Caffeine
COFFEE		
Brewed coffee (drip)	5 oz. cup	115
Brewed coffee (percolator)	5 oz. cup	80
Espresso (Starbucks)	1 oz. cup	89
Latte (Starbucks)	8 oz. cup	89
Cappuccino (Starbucks)	8 oz. cup	89
Instant coffee	5 oz. cup	65
Decaffeinated coffee	5 oz. cup	5
TEA		
Brewed tea	5 oz. cup	40
Snapple iced teas	16 oz. bottle	48
Decaffeinated tea	5 oz. cup	less than 5
Herbal teas	5 oz. cup	0
Iced tea	12 oz. glass	70
SOFT DRINKS		
Coca-Cola	12 oz.	45.6
Diet Coke	12 oz.	45.6
Pepsi-Cola	12 oz.	38.4
RC Cola	12 oz.	36
Jolt	12 oz.	71
Mountain Dew	12 oz.	55
Dr Pepper	12 oz.	39.6
Sunkist orange soda	12 oz.	40
Sprite	12 oz.	0
7UP	12 oz.	0
CHOCOLATES AND DESSERTS		
Dark chocolate (Hershey's)	1.5 oz.	31
Milk chocolate (Hershey's)	1.5 oz.	10
Baker's chocolate	1 oz.	26
1 Hershey's Kiss		1.2
Semisweet chocolate chips	1/4 cup	33

Food	Serving Size	Milligrams of Caffeine
Hot cocoa	8 oz.	5
Ben & Jerry's no-fat coffee-fudge frozen yogurt	1 cup	85
Starbucks coffee ice cream	1 cup	40–60
Dannon coffee yogurt	1 cup	45

Sources: U.S. Food and Drug Administration, Food Additive Chemistry Evaluation Branch; Center for Science in the Public Interest, Washington, D.C., 1998; Institute of Food Technologies, Washington, D.C., 1993, based on data from the National Soft Drink Association; data from the National Coffee Association; the Tea Council of the USA; and food and beverage labels and manufacturers.

chemotherapy drugs, and levodopa used to treat symptoms of Parkinson's disease. In rare cases, some women find oral contraceptives may interfere with sleep.

When talking about sleep problems with your doctor, be sure to discuss all medications, because you may not even be aware that some drugs can be stimulating. He or she may be able to prescribe alternative medications, or you may find you can take some medications in the morning instead of at night.

Resist Sleep Disrupters

Resist the temptation to use alcohol as a sleep aid. *Nightcap* is a misnomer. Alcohol may make you drowsy at first, but as it's metabolized two or three hours later, it wakes you up. Drinking before bedtime may also bring on morning headaches (or migraines) in women who are prone to them.

Alcohol alters the neurochemicals for sleep and mood and ultimately interferes with both. In general, it makes most things worse! Alcohol, even in small amounts, is sedating and may initially produce sleep, but it also alters the normal flow of sleep cycles. It retards the onset of REM sleep and may increase initial deep sleep. Once the alcohol is metabolized, a REM rebound will occur, and you'll awaken more easily. You're also likely to have rapid heartbeats and vivid dreams, which can disturb sleep. A chronic drinker or alcoholic can so alter her

Over-the-Counter Medications Containing Caffeine

Medication	Dose	Milligrams of Caffeine
ALERTNESS AIDS		
No-Doz (maximum strength)	1 tablet	200
No-Doz (regular strength)	1 tablet	100
Vivarin	1 tablet	100
PAIN RELIEVERS		
Excedrin	2 tablets	130
Anacin	2 tablets	64
Midol	2 tablets	64
PMS REMEDIES/DIURETICS		
Maximum strength Aqua-Ban Plus	1 tablet	200
Permathene H₂Off	1 tablet	200
Aqua-Ban	1 tablet	100
ALLERGY/COLD REMEDIES		
Coryban-D	1 capsule	30
Triaminic	1 tablet	30
Dristan	1 tablet	16
WEIGHT-CONTROL AIDS		
Dietac	1 capsule	200
Dexatrim	1 tablet	200
Prolamine	1 tablet	140
Maximum strength Appedrine	1 tablet	100

Source: U.S. Pharmacopeia, *Complete Drug Reference 1999* (Consumer Reports Books, FDA, National Center for Drugs and Biologics).

sleep mechanisms that she will find it virtually impossible to obtain good sleep for *years* after becoming sober. Insomnia is a huge problem for ex-alcoholics.

Alcohol can also change the physical aspects of one's sleep. As a sedative it dulls our response to decreased oxygen and increased carbon dioxide, so we may not breathe as well. It tends to swell nasal and oral

Prescription Medications That Interfere with Sleep

PRESCRIPTION DRUGS CONTAINING CAFFEINE

Drug	Dose (Tablets)	Milligrams of Caffeine
Cafergot (migraine reliever)	1	100
Fiorinal (headache reliever)	2	80
Fioricet (headache reliever)	2	80
Norgesic (muscle relaxant)	2	60
Darvon (pain reliever)	1	32

mucous membranes, so otherwise open noses and throats can get narrower, causing or worsening existing apnea. Nonsnorers may snore after a night of partying, and snorers may develop apnea. Those with apnea will have more severe episodes, cutting off the oxygen.

Besides its effect on respiration, alcohol can also worsen movement disorders like restless legs syndrome and periodic leg movements. Disorders of arousal such as sleepwalking or confused arousal increase because of the increase in deep sleep and the deadened ability to arouse thoroughly.

Alcohol also interferes with other hormones generated or balanced by sleep. These include melatonin, growth hormone, and serotonin. Therefore, alcohol has a negative effect on the timing of one's sleep rhythm as well as the sense of being refreshed by sleep. Regular nighttime drinkers will not be clearheaded or refreshed upon awakening and may be sluggish all morning; their performance may be off also. This typically leads to a cycle of repetition. You think, "Gee, I'm not sleeping well," so you increase the nightly alcohol to "get more sleep," and whammo, you're hooked. Any problem with sleep is increased, as is any sense of depression or anxiety.

It's also important to know that alcohol interferes with many other drugs you may be taking, particularly those for mood disorders. If you're using any antidepressant or other psychotherapeutic drug, skip the alcohol!

Resist recreational drugs. We all know they're not good for us, but

Other Medications That Can Affect Sleep

Class of Drug	Specific Drugs
Amphetamines	Dexedrine
Antidepressants	Monoamine oxidase inhibitors (e.g., Parnate, Nardil, Marplan)
	Selective serotonin reuptake inhibitors (e.g., Prozac, Zoloft, Paxil)
Antihypertensives	propanolol (Inderal)
Appetite suppressants	Fastin, Anorex
Brochodilators	theophylline, aminophylline, ephedrine
Cholesterol-lowering drugs	Lescor, Mevacor, Pravachol, Zocor
Corticosteroids (systemic)	Decadron, Hydrocortone, Meprolone, Prednisone
Ergot alkaloids (for headache)	Methylsergide
Parkinson's drugs (Levodopa)	Dopar, Larodopa, Sinemet,
Stimulants	ephedrine, methylphenidate (Ritalin)
Thyroid replacement hormones	levothyroxine (excess doses)

Source: U.S. Pharmacopeia, *Complete Drug Reference 1999* (Consumer Reports Books, FDA, National Center for Drugs and Biologics).

it's amazing how many adults (not silly adolescents, but adults) come to me insisting that their marijuana habit isn't interfering with their sleep. They believe they're medicating themselves to sleep! However, the active ingredient in marijuana alters sleep-related brain chemicals and triggers changes in brain wave patterns. In fact, long-term marijuana use can make it harder for you to get to sleep and reduce your REM sleep.

Morphine and heroin disrupt sleep, increasing muscle tension and awakenings. They also decrease the amounts of slow-wave and REM sleep. Although some tolerance to morphine can develop, chronic use leads to chronic insomnia. Methadone causes similar disturbances in sleep, but its chronic use doesn't lead to chronic insomnia.

Amphetamines can also interfere with sleep. They're initially stimulating and, of course, are used as legitimate medications to treat the sleep disorder of narcolepsy. They suppress REM sleep, which returns after a few days and rebounds significantly with withdrawal. Unfortunately, the "high" or increase in mood also significantly decreases with withdrawal and is probably what captures people into continued amphetamine use. Cocaine is a stimulant, which first makes you feel euphoric and energized; then you "crash." It is believed to have a similar effect on the sleep and wake systems.

Barbiturates, frequently used as sleeping pills, increase total sleep time and initially reduce REM sleep. They are seldom used for sleep today because we have many other, safer choices that are more targeted to act in the brain with fewer side effects over shorter periods of time.

Resist tobacco. Remember, nicotine is also a stimulant. Studies show women are more likely to turn to cigarettes to relieve stress. You may feel calmer after a smoke, but nicotine spurs production of the stress hormone adrenaline, which stimulates the brain as well as many other systems in the body. And while you're awake think about this: Smoking not only leads to high blood pressure, heart attacks, and strokes but also decreases normal estrogen production and speeds up bone loss (that's in addition to the increased risk of lung cancer). If you're chewing nicotine gum to stop smoking, try not to chew it after 3:00 in the afternoon.

Eat Right, Sleep Tight

When you eat, what you eat, and how much you eat are all very important in relation to the quality of your sleep. Again, keeping regular mealtimes helps maintain your biological clock.

Avoid heavy meals within four or five hours of bedtime (they can cause heartburn or worsen stomach acid reflux). Don't eat just before going to bed; instead opt for a light snack an hour or so before retiring. People who tend to eat their largest meal at night may consume many more calories than they would if they had eaten several meals across the day. This taxes the digestive system, which may have anticipated a shutdown, leading to weight gain as well.

Do I have a "recipe" for a sleep-inducing bedtime snack? Actually, I have several (see box on page 40).

Milk (warm or cold) contains the amino acid tryptophan, which converts in the brain to serotonin and helps modulate sleep (the process takes forty-five minutes to an hour). A glass of milk an hour or so before going to bed can help improve sleep onset and deepen sleep. It doesn't matter if it's nonfat or whole milk. Milk also provides extra calcium, which we all need to stave off bone loss.

Cheese, bananas, turkey, and even fish contain tryptophan. Combine them with a little carbohydrate to settle the stomach and promote sleep. Yes, the traditional milk and a cookie will do nicely (but just one or two, please).

I tell midlife women to make a bedtime milk shake with soy milk, silken tofu, or flavored soy protein powder (available in most health food stores), which some studies suggest may help quell hot flashes as well as aid sleep. Throw in a banana for the tryptophan. Add intense flavorings (decaf espresso), spices (like cinnamon and nutmeg), or extracts (like orange, lemon, almond, or vanilla) to help harmonize or overcome the distinct taste of soy and tofu products.

Noncaffeinated herbal teas are wonderfully soothing before bedtime. The herb valerian made as tea actually has some sedative properties and may help you sleep. Look for labels that say the product is "standardized" to contain 0.8 percent valeric acid (or valerenic acid); the generally accepted dose is 2 to 3 grams of dried root in tea, three times a day (the last cup thirty to forty-five minutes before bed). You can also take valerian in tablets or capsules, or as fluid extract or tincture (diluted in water). But don't use this herb for more than four to six weeks at a time. The taste is not everyone's cup of tea, however, so you might want to add honey. It takes two to three weeks of drinking valerian tea for it to become effective. Be warned, however, that valerian can cause dangerous interactions with benzodiazepines like alprazolam (Xanax), often prescribed as sleep aids. (For more on herbs, see pages 74–76.)

Watch your sugar and calories (especially if you crave fattening sweets during the premenstrual period). A big, gooey piece of chocolate cake with that glass of milk not only will sabotage your waistline but may also undermine your sleep because of the caffeine in the chocolate and

---

Three Sleep-Inducing Snacks

NIGHTLY NEWS MUNCH
4–5 whole grain crackers
1–2 oz. sliced turkey, cheese, or leftover tuna salad
8 oz. nonfat (or 1 percent) milk

BREAKFAST AT BEDTIME
1 sliced banana
1 cup high-fiber cold cereal
6 oz. nonfat (or 1 percent) milk
(1 tsp. ground soy nuts, optional)

SLEEPER SMOOTHIE
1 sliced banana
1–2 tsp. banana extract
$\frac{1}{2}$ cup fresh strawberries
Artificial sweetener (to taste)
$9\frac{1}{2}$ oz. ($\frac{1}{2}$ cake) silken tofu
$\frac{1}{4}$ cup soy milk
6 oz. nonfat (or 1 percent) milk
Blend in electric blender until creamy. Add more flavoring extract and milk if needed.

---

the high sugar content. If you eat a high-sugar snack before bedtime, you may experience a drop in blood sugar (glucose) while you sleep, and that can wake you up in the middle of the night!

Are You Ready for Some ZZZZZ's?

Now that you're familiar with some of the general features of sleep and sleep control, you can start to utilize these strategies to restore balance to your sleep and wake systems. The key is to know your situation and use these techniques properly. As a woman, be aware of your increased risk of sleep deprivation. The next few chapters will help you pinpoint your specific sleep problems and their solutions.

If you have a sleep disorder like narcolepsy, you may need medication or other measures. A complete discussion of sleep disorders and sleep medications can be found in Chapter 4. Sometimes a professional sleep clinician can help. It's frequently hard to sort out what the overriding problem is and choose—and use properly—the appropriate sleep aid. A rule of thumb is that if you have occasional problems sleeping, they're not likely to stem from a sleep disorder. If sleep problems are constant and last longer than a month, you may have an undiagnosed sleep disorder and may benefit from a session in the sleep lab (for more about this, see pages 164–65). By and large, however, armed with good information you'll be able to alleviate most of the sleep problems you'll encounter.

2

Our Raging Hormones

What's Keeping Us Awake?

More than half of the sleep problems we experience can be attributed to hormonal influences unique to us as females.

Not surprised, are you?

Whether you've been kept awake by menstrual cramps or hot flashes, you know that female hormones and the events governed by them exert a huge influence on our lives.

The National Sleep Foundation Women and Sleep Poll found that over 70 percent of menstruating women reported two and a half days of disrupted sleep during the premenstrual period; over a year that's the equivalent of almost a month spent tossing and turning! Most women complained about symptoms like bloating or breast tenderness, easily treated.

Almost 80 percent of pregnant women reported that their sleep was more disturbed during pregnancy. About a third found sleep was either longer or shorter, and 60 percent said that the sleep they did get was less refreshing. Menopausal or postmenopausal women reported more symptoms of insomnia than premenopausal women (56 versus 49 percent). Over a third of menopausal women said their sleep was interrupted by hot flashes *five* nights out of the week!

The likely culprit for these sleep disruptions is hormonal fluctuations. They're not the whole story, but let's examine their possible effects.

Your Hormones and Sleep Cycles

The same hormones that regulate our menstrual cycles and other processes in our bodies can influence the stages of sleep that I outlined in Chapter 1.

We know relatively little about *how* this occurs. Most of the studies of hormones and sleep have been done in animals, and *male* animals to boot! A few studies have been done recently in women, but they were small. Not all of them have taken into account the phases of the menstrual cycle. So it's hard to compare studies. Hey, it's hard to compare hormone levels within an individual woman; they're seldom the same from month to month. Still, we do have some good ideas about how hormones influence sleep. And this interaction frames sleep problems in a different way: a hormonal imbalance we can often *do* something about.

So what's a hormone, you may ask? *Hormones* are defined as substances or chemicals produced by a gland, an organ (including the brain), or a tissue that regulates specific body functions. Hormones secreted by one gland can affect other glands or organs and interact with one another. An abnormality in one hormone may set off a chain reaction in a variety of systems. A good example is thyroid hormone. Although the thyroid is primarily responsible for regulating metabolism, too much thyroid hormone can cause irregular heartbeats, bone loss, anxiety, and sleep disruption. Too little can cause weight gain, dry skin, infertility, excess sleepiness, and depression.

Remember our seesaw and balls? They may be in perfect balance until we add the influence of hormones. Now, picture those two balls full of bouncing bubbles that fly back and forth on their own schedules, sometimes filling one ball, sometimes the other. That's what happens with fluctuating hormones.

Think of how your moods can fluctuate; hormones are involved in them, too. Sleep and mood involve the same major chemical messengers in the brain (called neurotransmitters): serotonin and norepinephrine. Serotonin can affect mood, sleep, pain, even appetite (and that's the short list). Norepinephrine is triggered in response to stress.

With me so far?

Now we come to sex hormones. It's important to remember that male and female sex hormones are present in both sexes, just in different amounts. Our adrenal glands secrete small amounts of male hormones (androgens), as do the ovaries. Women, of course, have more estrogen and less testosterone than men, but we need male hormones, too (they're actually converted to estrogen in the brain). Some of this testosterone is also stored in fat, muscles, and other tissues and converted there to estrogen. Estrogen regulates our menstrual cycles and helps maintain many tissues and organs, including bones; progesterone plays an important role in the menstrual cycle and pregnancy.

So, how do these sex hormones factor into sleep?

As I mentioned in Chapter 1, women have more deep, slow-wave sleep than men and a slower age-related decline in deep sleep than men. Many researchers believe female hormones play a role in this. Brain cells, including those areas involved in the sleep-wake cycle, have receptors for sex hormones. Exogenous hormones (those we take in birth control pills and hormone replacement) also affect sleep. Researchers find that estrogen seems to enhance REM sleep (decreasing the time it takes to get to dream sleep and increasing the amount of REM sleep). Estrogen replacement also seems to increase slow-wave sleep after menopause, lessening the age-related decline.

As for progesterone, every sleep study shows that it seems to have a sedating effect, almost in the same way a sleeping pill would. Progesterone appears to reduce the amount of time it takes to get to sleep and the number of episodes of wakefulness after we get to sleep. When administered intravenously, progesterone increases NREM sleep.

Testosterone has different effects on sleep in men and women (remember, testosterone is converted to estrogen in the brain). In males, testosterone decreases REM sleep. But since we have slightly more REM sleep than men well into our sixties, it's not so much the total quantity of testosterone that matters. What's important for us is the balance between female and male hormones.

After menopause, when the ovaries start shutting down and estrogen declines, that balance changes, because testosterone is made mostly in the adrenals, not the ovaries. We don't produce *more* testosterone (levels actually fall), but the ratio of testosterone to estrogen is higher. (Contrary to popular belief, we're never totally out of estrogen even after menopause. Other forms of estrogen are still produced in fatty tissues and elsewhere.)

Women sensitive to the effects of androgens will feel this hormonal shift acutely, with symptoms of irritability, sleeplessness, and depression similar to those caused by estrogen loss. Because testosterone also helps regulate the sex drive, lower levels of this hormone after menopause can cause libido to take a nosedive. Adding back small amounts of testosterone not only can help libido but may also improve some mood and sleep problems. Replacing estrogen can also help sleep.

Estrogen also regulates the flow of other key hormones that are secreted during sleep, among them growth hormone, prolactin, cortisol, and melatonin. (This starts to get a little technical, but bear with me.)

Growth hormone (gH), secreted by the pituitary, is needed throughout life for growth development, and repair of body tissues, and it is secreted early in the night, at the onset of sleep. Maybe that's why Mom told you you needed to get your sleep to grow! When the timing and duration of deep sleep change, so does the secretion of growth hormone. We have less growth hormone as we get older, and we spend less time in deep sleep. Premenopausal women have higher levels of growth hormone than men, and gH levels appear most elevated during the premenstrual period.

Cortisol also stimulates slow-wave sleep and production of growth hormone through a feedback loop, rising in the late morning and early afternoon, decreasing in the evening. In people with depression, cortisol is elevated all the time.

Prolactin (PRL) is also produced by the pituitary under the influence of estrogen. This hormone is secreted in waves, or pulses, during sleep. But it has a circadian rhythm all its own, governed by our biological clocks. Women have more prolactin than men, and its pattern of secretion has been linked to increased slow-wave sleep. Production of prolactin is greatly affected by the environment, light, stress, meals, even sexual activity.

Melatonin is known as the hormone of darkness, because it is produced by the pineal gland at night and is thought to have a role in regulating sleep. Production of melatonin can also be increased by estrogen. Together they may influence our response to other stress hormones. Later on, I'll discuss how this interaction may also influence moods during the menstrual cycle. In people with seasonal affective disorder, a form of depression related to changing patterns of daylight and darkness, levels of melatonin are found to increase during the winter months, causing daytime sleepiness and longer periods of sleep.

We believe that melatonin's effects on sleep may come through body temperature. Remember, we're more likely to fall asleep when our body temperature is falling and wake as it rises. Melatonin lowers body temperature. A number of drugs, among them aspirin, ibuprofen, and high blood pressure medications called beta blockers, as well as alcohol, nicotine, and caffeine (which may be among the reasons cigarettes and coffee cause wakefulness), may suppress melatonin secretion.

By now, you've gotten the idea that the relationship of hormones to sleep is a complex one. Our sleep seesaw can be bounced up and down like crazy by the effects of these various hormones at different points in our menstrual cycles and in our lives.

Our Childbearing (Menstrual) Years

We can divide the menstrual cycle into four phases: the menstruation phase, which starts on day 1 of the cycle with the onset of our period; the follicular phase, which leads up to ovulation (which usually occurs around day 14); the early luteal phase, which covers the week or so after ovulation (days 15 to 21); and the late luteal phase, which follows until menstruation starts again (days 22 to 28). Each phase can be determined by the levels of circulating hormones. Remember those bubbles crossing between the balls on the seesaw? For some women the menstrual years feel like bouncing bubbles. It's no wonder, so many hormones are involved!

In the follicular phase the brain signals the pituitary gland to produce a surge of follicle-stimulating hormone (FSH), which triggers increased estrogen production and stimulates follicles in the ovaries. At midcycle a surge of luteinizing hormone (LH) causes one of the follicles to burst open and release a mature egg. The egg is gathered into the fallopian tubes, where it must be fertilized within six to eight hours or it will begin to deteriorate. The shell of the follicle becomes the corpus luteum, which produces progesterone. (In Latin, *corpus luteum* means "yellow body"; the spent follicle actually leaves a yellow pockmark on the ovary.)

Ovulation occurs right after the LH surge. During the luteal phase of the cycle, LH levels fall as the corpus luteum produces more progesterone, which, with estrogen, stimulates growth of the top layer of a blanket of blood vessels and nutrients inside the uterus to prepare for the implantation of a fertilized egg. Progesterone levels peak about seven days after ovulation. If the egg is not fertilized, the corpus luteum degenerates and progesterone levels drop. The uterine lining breaks up and is shed as menstrual flow. This ovulatory-menstrual cycle typically lasts between twenty-six and thirty-two days, although women can have shorter or longer cycles.

So how does the menstrual cycle influence our sleep? During menstruation most of our hormone secretion lessens, as does our metabolic rate. As a result, many women experience excessive daytime sleepiness. In rare cases women suffer hypersomnia, excessive daytime sleepiness that begins premenstrually and clears up after a period arrives. This may be the result of sensitivity to progesterone's sedating effects.

Studies by Dr. Helen Driver, a sleep researcher at the University Health Network, Toronto, with colleagues at the University of Zurich, suggest that in the follicular phase, as estrogen production begins to rise, many women experience an increased amount of stage 2 and sleep spindles. We can expect an increase in REM sleep, too, in response to the action of estrogen during the follicular phase.

During the early luteal phase, progesterone begins to rise and acts to increase body temperature and blunt the circadian rhythm. Over the next fourteen days, we'll have increased wakefulness and increased sleep disturbance. We tend to get sleepy earlier and wake up earlier because our melatonin rhythm is blunted. Our metabolic rate increases as well. We also experience a decrease in the depth of sleep and an increase in the time it takes to fall asleep.

Some studies have also reported that in the late luteal phase, when estrogen and progesterone levels fall, women have more nighttime awakenings and a greater percentage of NREM sleep. Dr. Driver and other researchers find a significant decrease in slow-wave sleep premenstrually, decreased sleep efficiency, increase in the time it takes to fall asleep, and decreased sleep quality.

For women who experience premenstrual syndrome (PMS), these symptoms may be worse. Premenstrual syndrome varies from woman to woman. Clinically, it's defined as a group of symptoms that arise in the period between ovulation and menstruation. Researchers theorize that some women have a special sensitivity to normal hormonal (or physical) changes in the luteal phase of their cycle, which may trigger symptoms. A small study at the National Institute of Mental Health in 1998 suggested that PMS symptoms stem from abnormal reactions in the brain to female hormones. Researchers suppressed the menstrual cycles of twenty women (half of whom had PMS), then added back estrogen, progesterone, or a placebo. Only those women with PMS reported PMS-like symptoms when given hormones. That's as close as anyone's come in finding biological clues about PMS.

More than a hundred symptoms, including fluid retention, bloating, weight gain, headaches, acne, breast tenderness, and cravings for sweets or carbohydrates, as well as depression, anxiety, irritability, mood swings, tearfulness, and changes in sex drive, are associated with PMS. Women with added life stress may find that the quality of their sleep declines. They may also experience daytime sleepiness and increased sleep disturbances.

Some women have PMS from their first menstrual period on, but women are more likely to develop it during their thirties and forties, especially after pregnancy or stopping use of the birth control pill. Many women develop PMS during perimenopause, when hormones fluctuate wildly.

That's what hormone studies say. What do women say?

Women indeed report the most sleep disruptions just before menstruation and at the start of menstrual flow, when estrogen and progesterone are lowest. In the National Sleep Foundation survey, 73 percent of menstruating women reported that their sleep was affected by cramping, bloating, headaches, and tender breasts during the week before their periods. The most common complaint was bloating, reported by 50 percent of women premenstrually and 25 percent after their periods began. It is interesting that more women reported disturbed sleep caused by menstrual cycle factors during the first days of their periods (71 percent) than in the week before (43 percent).

Of those women whose sleep was most disturbed during the week before or during the first few days of their period, 51 percent reported taking longer to fall asleep. Forty-one percent woke more often during the night and had a hard time getting back to sleep, and more than half awoke earlier in the morning and awoke feeling less refreshed than during the rest of the month.

You can see a correlation between what researchers have learned about the effects of hormones on sleep during the menstrual cycle and the disturbances women are reporting.

Premenstrual Mood and Sleep Problems

Some researchers believe that symptoms of PMS, especially sleep problems, may be caused by circadian rhythm disturbances.

According to research by Dr. Sally Severino, former vice chair of psychiatry at the University of New Mexico Health Sciences Center, and Dr. Margaret Moline, director of the Sleep-Wake Disorders Center at the Westchester campus of the New York Presbyterian Hospital, women who suffer PMS may complain of nighttime sleep disturbances and daytime sleepiness, with mood changes and difficulty concentrating, not unlike what happens to shift workers and jet-lagged travelers.

It's possible that these temporary problems may involve shifts in the secretion of melatonin. Its usual rhythm is low blood levels during the day and high blood levels at night. Melatonin may also modulate the menstrual cycle, and it has been found to be higher premenstrually and during menstruation. The National Sleep Foundation survey found that 68 percent of menstruating women felt sleepiest during the week before or the first few days of their periods, compared with the rest of the month. Melatonin (along with progesterone) may have something to do with this. It's a still unproven theory that's under active study.

Dr. Moline believes low serotonin is a likely culprit. In addition to physical symptoms and sleep problems, many women have cravings for sweets or carbohydrates, which many researchers link to low serotonin

---

PMDD Checklist

To meet the diagnosis for premenstrual dysphoric disorder, you must have five (or more) of the following symptoms most of the time during the luteal phase of most of your menstrual cycles. Symptoms should subside a few days after your period starts.

- Noticeable depressed mood, feelings of hopelessness, worthlessness
- Feeling of being overwhelmed or out of control
- Heightened anxiety and tension
- Marked mood swings (feeling suddenly sad, irritable, or angry)
- Persistent anger or irritability, increased interpersonal conflicts
- Decreased interest in normal activities
- Difficulty concentrating
- Lethargy and fatigue
- Change in appetite (overeating or food cravings)
- Sleeping too much or trouble sleeping
- Physical symptoms such as breast tenderness, headaches, bloating, joint or muscle pain, weight gain

Source: *Diagnostic and Statistical Manual of Mental Disorders,* 4th edition *(DSM-IV),* American Psychiatric Press, 1994.

---

levels. Low serotonin may also contribute to PMS-related mood swings, depression, and anxiety.

Some women suffer an especially severe mood problem called *premenstrual dysphoric disorder* (PMDD). This is primarily a disorder of mood (though the physical symptoms of PMS may be present). One of the hallmarks of PMDD is sleep problems.

Premenstrual dysphoric disorder actually has the features of major depression, but it occurs only during the week or two before menstruation. Symptoms are tracked with daily diaries kept for at least two cycles. For a diagnosis, a woman must experience these symptoms during most of her menstrual cycles severely enough to interfere with school or work and social or marital relationships.

So, what do we think is going on with hormones in PMDD? Major depression has been linked to disruptions in the hypothalamic-pituitary-

Fighting Bloat, Finding Hidden Salt

Bloating is the number-one PMS complaint and a sleep robber; a major cause is salt. But even if you banish the saltshaker from the table, you'll still be getting plenty of sodium hidden in foods. And many of us are sensitive to sodium and retain fluid, especially before our periods.

Steer clear of high-sodium seasonings like soy sauce or ketchup. Instead, try seasonings with little or no salt, such as fresh herbs, spices, vinegar, or lemon juice. Even so-called salt substitutes may contain sodium. Read product labels. Reduced or "light" products have half the amount of sodium, but that may still be considerable.

Ninety percent of prepared or processed foods, such as cold cuts, pickles, and potato chips, contain high amounts of sodium. Even an otherwise healthy salad may contain 237 milligrams of sodium in 2 tablespoons of bottled Italian dressing. Here's a brief list of high-sodium foods.

FOODS HIGH IN SODIUM

Food Choices	Milligrams of Sodium
Sauerkraut: canned, juice, 1 cup	1904
Pickle: dill, 1 large (4 inches)	1827
Soup, canned: Manhattan clam chowder, 1 cup*	1827
Bouillon: chicken, from cube, 1 cup*	1536
Ham: boneless, roasted, 3 oz.	1177
Soy sauce: regular, 1 T	1029
Potato chips*	950
Tuna: canned, in oil, 3 oz.*	930
Tomato juice: canned or bottled, 1 cup*	878
Olives: green, 10	827
Broth: canned, beef or chicken, 1 cup*	780
Pork and Beans: canned, 1 cup**	770
Pretzels: salted, 1 cup*	756
Bacon: Canadian style, 2 slices	719
Sausage: kielbasa, 1 oz.	687
Pizza: 12-inch cheese with regular crust, 1/4 pie	673
Turkey cold cuts: 2 slices*	608
Spaghetti sauce: jar, 1/2 cup*	500

Food Choices	Milligrams of Sodium
Hot dog: beef, 1*	461
Processed American cheese spread, 1 oz.	461
Pudding: powdered, prepared w/ whole milk, 1/2 cup*	410

*Average sodium content for product of this type.
**In general, commercial canned vegetables contain an average of 500 milligrams of sodium per cup, unless labeled low-sodium.

Source: U.S. Department of Agriculture; National Heart, Lung, and Blood Institute

adrenal (HPA) axis, which regulates production of stress hormones like cortisol and norepinephrine (remember those?). Some studies show that norepinephrine activity increases shortly before ovulation and continues through the luteal phase; high norepinephrine levels are associated with anxiety and decreased ability to sleep. The HPA axis is also affected by pregnancy (a possible clue to postpartum depression, see pages 94–95). The other mood- and sleep-related chemical, serotonin, is also found to be lower during the luteal phase, especially in women who suffer from premenstrual depression. (Remember that estrogen and progesterone interact with the same chemicals that control mood.) It's also known that progesterone, which is increased during the premenstrual period, has depressive effects. The antidepressant fluoxetine (Prozac) has been approved for the treatment of PMDD.

Put all of this together with what we know about hormones and sleep, and you can see the possible connections. Researchers are now trying to confirm them.

Sleep Problems During Pregnancy

A majority of the pregnant women surveyed by the National Sleep Foundation reported that their sleep was more disturbed during pregnancy, and over half said their sleep was less refreshing.

Why is that?

The placenta produces high levels of many hormones, including estrogen, progesterone, and prolactin. Progesterone is often called the

Your Sleep Rx for PMS

You can do many things to relieve your PMS symptoms and lessen sleep problems. Because bloating seems to be a major sleep disrupter, avoid salty foods, especially if you're salt-sensitive, since they can cause you to retain fluid. If your fingers seem swollen and your rings get tight after you've eaten a pickle or a bag of salted potato chips, chances are you're sensitive to sodium. When you have the munchies, go for unsalted snacks. Beware of hidden salt in processed foods and seasonings (see the box on pages 51–52).

• Drink lots of water. Paradoxically, water is a diuretic; the more we drink, the more we may be able to flush our system of excess sodium (which makes us retain fluid).

• If your bloating is severe and is causing nighttime discomfort, prescription diuretics such as chlorthalidone (Hygroton), furosemide (Lasix), and hydrochlorothiazide (HydroDIURIL) can help the kidneys get rid of excess salt and water and reduce fluid retention. An over-the-counter product combining ammonium chloride and caffeine (such as Aqua-Ban) has less diuretic action, but it also relieves bloating and is a mild stimulant. Other over-the-counter remedies like Midol contain acetaminophen, caffeine, and pyrilamine maleate (a diuretic). Dandelion herb tea is regarded as a natural diuretic. Drink it three to four times a day; you need 4 to 10 grams of the herb a day to relieve PMS symptoms. Don't take any diuretic in the evening or you'll spend the night in the bathroom, and those with caffeine may also interfere with sleep.

• Take extra calcium. A recent study at Columbia University among five hundred women found that those who took 1,200 milligrams of calcium carbonate (in the form of Tums, which paid for the study) reduced premenstrual symptoms by 50 percent. Bloating and water retention was cut by 36 percent, psychological symptoms were reduced by 45 percent, and food cravings dropped by

54 percent. There are now candylike calcium chews (such as Viac-
tiv) that have a double benefit: You get 500 milligrams of calcium
carbonate and 100 international units of vitamin D with each cube.
They are also a great way to satisfy your cravings for sweets (most
chews have 15 to 20 calories per cube).

Calcium may even have a slightly sedative effect, so it's not a bad
idea to take your supplements right after dinner. (Combine your
calcium with magnesium to help with leg cramps and insomnia; the
combination seems to act like a muscle relaxant.) But too much
calcium can lead to kidney stones or other health problems, so
check with your doctor about a recommended daily dose.

• Try extra magnesium. Another recent study suggests that
PMS symptoms may be linked to low blood levels of magnesium.
The researchers believe low levels of magnesium may affect the
secretion of neurochemicals (like serotonin) that affect mood and
also lead to dilation of blood vessels that cause bloating. The recommended daily allowance of magnesium is 400 milligrams; many
multivitamins contain only a fraction of that. You can get extra
magnesium from supplements and from foods like nuts, bran,
whole wheat bread, green leafy vegetables, and fruit. Ask your doctor to recommend a maximum daily dosage.

• A 1999 review of nine clinical trials involving more than nine
hundred women reported in the *British Medical Journal* found that
100 milligrams of vitamin B_6 (pyridoxine) daily helped ease symptoms of PMS. Taking more than 200 milligrams a day can cause
damage to nerves. It's important to remember that vitamins are
drugs, too. Megadoses of certain vitamins can be toxic. Check with
your doctor before taking any vitamins or other supplements.

• Don't eat too many sweets. High-sugar foods and drinks can
disturb sleep. Sugar is quickly metabolized, so you can suffer a sudden drop in blood sugar that will wake you up.

Speaking of sweets, we all know that chocolate makes us feel good and increases serotonin and dopamine levels. But chocolate *does* contain caffeine, fat, and calories. So eat no more than 2 ounces of dark chocolate close to bedtime (that would give you as much caffeine as a cup of coffee), and no more than 3 ounces of milk chocolate (it has less caffeine but more fat).

• Avoid coffee and other caffeinated beverages. Not only can they keep you awake but they also increase anxiety and irritability (and may contribute to breast tenderness). See the chart on caffeine on pages 33–34.

• Limit alcohol; as women we may be more sensitive to its effects (and have higher blood levels of alcohol per ounce of liquor) premenstrually. And, as I've mentioned, alcohol disrupts the structure of sleep.

• If you're experiencing major trouble falling asleep premenstrually, ask your physician for something to help you sleep those few days a month. The new sleep aid zaleplon (Sonata) may be especially helpful because it can be used as needed and is short-acting.

• Try herbs and herbal preparations (with my caveats on pages 75–76). A blend of almond oil and chamomile is a very good antispasmodic that some women rub on their bellies to ease cramps. Primrose oil, available in capsules, has been found to be helpful in relieving PMS symptoms because it has anti-inflammatory properties. But don't take more than 3 grams a day; if you have stomachaches and diarrhea, you may be taking too much. Chaste tree fruit extract is also good for PMS and breast pain (see herb chart on pages 78–80). Ginger tea may help menstrual cramps. Ginseng can ease fatigue, depression, and stress. I can't emphasize enough, however, that herbs are not regulated and doses are not standardized. What's "natural" isn't always safe, so check with your doctor before taking any herbs.

• Try some stress busters (see pages 30–31) as alternative remedies for PMS-related irritability and mood swings.

• Use heat and cold. A heating pad often helps relieve cramping. Ice packs are useful for breast tenderness, along with an extra 400 milligrams of vitamin E a day.

• Launch a preemptive strike against pain. Nonsteroidal anti-inflammatory drugs (NSAIDs), like aspirin, ibuprofen, and keto-profen, suppress substances in the body called prostaglandins, which cause menstrual cramps. Take them before you go to bed to avoid midsleep awakenings brought on by cramping. Aceta-minophen has no effect on prostaglandins and won't help menstrual cramps. However, it can be good for muscle aches. A sleep aid combining acetaminophen (such as Tylenol PM) with the anti-histamine diphenhydramine (which makes some people drowsy) will help you get a good night's rest if you have other aches and pains that keep you awake.

• Exercise can help relieve PMS symptoms, and it promotes a good night's sleep. But, again, try to avoid strenuous exercise within two to three hours of bedtime.

hormone of pregnancy, and, while it has sedating effects, many other things occur during those nine months that interfere with sleep. For example, a woman may have nausea and vomiting, backaches, leg cramps, and heartburn, not to mention the need to urinate more often and the baby kicking while she's trying to sleep. She may have more frequent nightmares during pregnancy and suffer from breathing problems, including sleep apnea (which causes frequent awakenings during the night).

Pregnancy hormones also cause connective tissues to soften (to accommodate the growing belly and its strains on the body). The joints between the pelvic bones also become more relaxed to allow the baby to pass through during delivery. However, this can cause hip pain, usually

---

Getting the Most from Calcium

We need calcium to build bone mass when we're young and prevent bone loss later in life. Most women don't know that calcium can also promote better sleep. But study after study shows that women are not getting the calcium they need. The average woman only gets *half* of the recommended 1,200 milligrams of calcium a day before menopause, and the minimum of 1,500 milligrams after menopause. You also need 400 international units a day of vitamin D to help calcium absorption.

The forms of calcium that are broken down and used most easily by the body are calcium citrate (used to fortify orange juice) and calcium carbonate (the form in Tums and Rolaids). Calcium citrate has a slight edge. A 1999 report that looked at fifteen studies on how well calcium carbonate and calcium citrate were absorbed by the body found a 22 to 27 percent greater absorption of calcium citrate. On the downside, calcium citrate is more expensive.

Calcium gluconate, calcium phosphate, calcium malate, and chelated calcium are fairly easily absorbed, oyster shell calcium less so. Look for the "USP" on the label; the United States Pharmacopoeia seal guarantees that each tablet contains the specified amount of elemental calcium. You should take two to three doses of 600 milligrams each, preferably with meals, during the day or evening.

But don't rely totally on supplements. Of course, dairy foods are your best source of calcium (look for low-fat or nonfat choices), but fish like canned salmon or sardines, green leafy vegetables like kale or collard greens, soybeans, nuts, sesame seeds, calcium-fortified fruit juices, and even mineral water are also good sources of calcium. And don't overdo it; taking too much calcium can lead to problems such as kidney stones.

---

on one side, in the third trimester. Changes in posture can also cause pain in the lower back.

One study of pregnant women found that 67 percent experienced backaches at night, and over a third complained that back pain awakened them. Sixty percent of the women said leg cramps disturbed their sleep.

Let's look at sleep in each trimester of pregnancy.

Foods High in Magnesium

Food Choices	Milligrams of Magnesium
VEGETABLES	
Spinach: fresh, cooked—1/2 cup	79
Chard: cooked, 1/2 cup	76
Beans, lima: cooked, 1/2 cup	63
Broccoli: cooked, 1/2 cup	47
Okra: cooked, 1/2 cup	46
Squash, acorn: cooked, 1/2 cup	43
BREADS, CEREALS, AND OTHER GRAINS	
All-Bran cereal, 1 oz.	106
Wheat germ: plain, 1 oz.	91
Bran Buds cereal, 1 oz.	90
BEANS/ LEGUMES (DRIED)	
Soybeans: green, cooked, 1/2 cup	54
Beans: white, black, or brown, dry, cooked, 1/2 cup	52–60
NUTS AND SEEDS	
Pumpkin or squash seeds: hulled, 1 oz.	152
Watermelon seeds, 1 oz.	146
Sunflower seeds: hulled, unroasted, 1 oz.	100
Almonds: roasted, dry roasted, or unroasted, 1 oz.	86
Filberts (or hazelnuts), 1 oz.	85
MILK/YOGURT	
Milk: skim, 1 cup	36
Yogurt: plain, low-fat, 4 oz.	19.8
SEAFOOD	
Clams: raw	55
Scallops: baked/broiled/boiled, 3 oz.	42

Source: U.S. Department of Agriculture

THE FIRST TRIMESTER

Sleep problems during the first trimester initially have to do with excessive sleepiness, thought to be caused by the rapid rise of progesterone during the initial weeks of pregnancy. Progesterone can cause as much daytime sleepiness as a sleeping pill. In fact, many women in this trimester are unable to stay awake during the day.

However, as pregnancy progresses, women begin to suffer from increased insomnia. Dr. Kathryn Lee, a sleep researcher at the University of California, San Francisco, notes that women's sleep becomes disrupted as early as eleven weeks into pregnancy, with increased awakenings, a shorter time to fall asleep, and less efficient sleep. Some studies show a slight decline in REM and slow-wave sleep, perhaps because of more awakenings.

Even before the expanding uterus begins to press on the bladder, women start having to make more frequent trips to the bathroom. This may also have to do with progesterone's inhibitory effects on smooth muscle contraction (the bladder walls and urethra are made of smooth muscle tissue). Some women may also be bothered at night by nausea (which is hormone-related), breast tenderness, and the aforementioned backaches.

THE SECOND TRIMESTER

During the second trimester, sleep actually improves, as though all our body systems have adjusted to the new developments and are on an even keel. However, many women are bothered by fetal movements and the emergence of pregnancy-related heartburn. Dr. Lee's studies show that women in the second trimester have more fragmented sleep and less deep sleep (stages 3–4) than they did before pregnancy.

Restless leg activity may also start during the second trimester. This is that creepy, crawly feeling that prompts you to move your legs to relieve the annoying sensations. Frequently, the feelings increase with fatigue and relaxation. (For more on restless legs, see pages 145–46.) Yes, the leg movements that seem to bother pregnant women do clear up after pregnancy.

THE THIRD TRIMESTER

The third trimester is a time of increasing sleep difficulty, in part because of the girth of the body and the inability to be comfortable and in part because of hormones changing before delivery. Sleep deprivation and fatigue are major issues late in the third trimester.

Women also suffer from shortness of breath, frequent urination, cramps, itching, and frequent nightmares. And heartburn increases along with the size of the belly. Frequent small meals, elevating the head of your bed, and avoiding spicy foods are especially important during this period.

The growing uterus also can press on the sciatic nerve (there are two of them, which run from the lower back down each leg), causing pain. Vaginal pain may be caused by the cervix's beginning to dilate.

The sleep-robbing anxiety that comes with feeling overwhelmed is a common problem at this time (and higher levels of hormones don't help). The other day while walking home, I saw a young couple (a very pregnant woman and her husband) with two small children in tow walk out of a nearby park. She was clearly angry, and he was trying to placate her. "You don't understand, of course I care about your needs and the kids, but I'm tired. You could have taken the kids to the park by yourself today. I didn't have to go, I could have taken a nap," she was saying. "You can do the laundry as well as I can. If you want a nice dinner, let's order out. I just need sleep. I can't sleep!"

She was typical of many women in this state. How do we sleep well with a huge belly, with its accompanying indigestion, worries about when and how delivery will occur, and on top of that, the responsibilities of children and family? I couldn't make it better for that woman, but you can make it better for yourself.

Realize that pregnancy can be a time of increased anxiety and do as much as possible to reduce stress. I recommend that you use deep breathing and relaxation exercises, ask your partner for soothing massages, and give yourself plenty of minivacations from everyday chores. Anything from a facial or manicure to a weekend away in a hotel (if that's in your budget). Don't ask for, *demand* extra help from your partner. Sit down, relax, and put your feet up as often as you can; your ankles will be swollen, and you need the break. Choose foods that aid sleep (more about this in a moment).

I also want to mention one other sleep-related problem that could crop up in late pregnancy. Because of the increasing size of the fetus (with the ballooning uterus pressing on the diaphragm) and shifting hormones, you may develop temporary sleep apnea (see Chapter 4). If you begin to snore or show other symptoms, like excessive daytime sleepiness, tell your doctor. Don't let your physician dismiss these complaints. The apnea could be interfering with the oxygen levels vital for the baby's growth. A simple oximetry test (done with a gadget you put on your finger during sleep) can monitor your oxygen during the night. (This is not the same thing as *fetal* pulse oximetry, and will not harm the baby.) This is a specialized reading, which prints out the entire night's oxygen levels (not just averaging it). If this test reveals frequent drops in oxygen during the night, ask for a referral to a sleep laboratory. A CPAP (continuous positive airway pressure) mask worn at night for the rest of your pregnancy will protect you and your baby.

The Postpartum Period

During the postpartum period, when our hormones are settling back to normal, so are our neurotransmitters, which control mood and sleep. Research shows that there's actually little change in the amount or structure of sleep between the immediate postpartum period and the late stages of pregnancy. But we hardly need mention the famed sleep loss caused by the interruptions required for feeding the new baby during the night and the stresses of new motherhood (see Chapter 3).

Sleep loss is a major culprit in mood problems and in the memory loss of new mothers (which may also be hormone-related). First-time mothers are especially at risk for postpartum depression (see Chapter 3), simply because they have no firsthand experience to draw on for coping with the increased stress. First-time moms also show a significant decrease in sleep efficiency and increase in fatigue compared with women who have more children. While the responsibilities and fears related to new motherhood can be staggering, don't forget that hor-

mones are bubbling again, whether you're adjusting to nursing or settling down into a regular rhythm. You may feel hyperalert at night
instead of sleepy.

Most of the sleep disturbance following childbirth occurs in the first
two to three months and involves difficulty initiating and maintaining
sleep. Dr. Pat Coble, a sleep researcher at the Western Psychiatric Institute of the University of Pittsburgh, suggests that the sleep systems of
women with histories of depression may be more sensitive to the psy-
chobiological changes of childbearing and that they may have earlier
onset or more severe sleep disruption.

Some research suggests that the "baby blues," those ups and downs
of mood we have after delivery, are actually the results of hormones acting on a brain center designed to make us keenly aware of the baby and
its needs, to help us better care for our baby. This may also cause us to
be hyperalert at night, aware of the baby's every movement, for some
women causing sleep loss and sleep fragmentation. (For some women,
having their baby sleeping close by may promote more peaceful sleep,
while others simply can't sleep with a bassinet at the bedside. There's no
"right" way; do what feels right for *you*.)

This is an intriguing theory. According to Dr. Laura Miller, a psychiatrist at the University of Illinois at Chicago, the "baby blues" may be
a *normal* state of heightened reactivity, similar to biological attachment
systems seen in animals. In such systems hormonal triggers create
heightened responses to stimuli in certain brain circuits, activating
maternal behavior. These hormones also affect the limbic system, the
center of our emotions.

One of the hormones involved in this postpartum reactivity is oxytocin (a pituitary hormone that triggers uterine contractions in labor and
the release of milk during lactation). Oxytocin increases at about thirty-
six weeks of pregnancy (a full-term pregnancy is forty weeks). This hormone, along with the rapid drop in estrogen and progesterone after
delivery and reactions from other neurochemicals, may promote mood
swings and anxiety. This knowledge casts sleep fragmentation and the
baby blues in a whole different light, doesn't it? However, we're not
talking about postpartum depression here. That's a separate issue. If

you've had a previous episode of major depression, you're at much higher risk for postpartum depression and may need to take preventive steps with medication.

For some women breast feeding is very soothing and relaxing. For others it's a pain, quite literally. It's your call. The baby gets the most benefit from breast milk in the first six weeks or so. Don't forget we benefit, too (faster uterine healing, the exquisite bonding that takes place, plus no periods). You can always express milk and have your partner take over night feedings. If leaky breasts are a problem, wear your nursing bra to bed with clean pads. However, if you find that breast feeding is making you crazy—stop! The baby will be okay, and your friends and family will just have to deal with it. It's your baby, your breast, your sleep, and your decision.

Some women do have hot flashes and night sweats right after delivery because of a drop in estrogen, which may continue during breast feeding. Follow the tips on page 77 for coping with this temporary annoyance.

The important thing is to remember that life is life, and this period of adjustment to changing hormones, motherhood, and babies' schedules doesn't last forever. We adapt, and we have to give ourselves time and permission to be a little cranky while doing so. Let's indulge ourselves, but let's not overdo it. I definitely think the late-night trips to the fridge should be discouraged by keeping a bowl of hard, sugarless candy by the bed, with water or juice in a nearby thermos. Why make another bad habit we only have to break?

Sleep and Assisted Reproduction

Women who are trying to become pregnant, by either artificial insemination or in vitro fertilization, should be aware that the high doses of hormones needed to stimulate the ovaries to release more than one egg can interfere with sleep.

The most commonly used fertility drug, clomiphene citrate (Clomid, Serophene), tricks the pituitary gland into producing more luteinizing hormone (LH) and follicle-stimulating hormone (FSH). It's taken orally for five days each month, so ovulation will occur by day 14 of the cycle. It can trigger higher production of progesterone and lengthen the luteal phase of the cycle. So you may experience more severe PMS-like symptoms, especially mood swings, bloating, and breast tenderness. It can also cause hot flashes. Human menopausal gonadotropins or hMGs (Pergonal, Repronex, Humegon) also cause PMS-like symptoms.

Gonadotropin-releasing hormone agonists (GnRH agonists) suppress follicle-stimulating hormone and luteinizing hormone (FSH and LH), so stimulation of the ovaries can be tightly controlled with other drugs for in vitro fertilization. These drugs throw women into a pseudomenopause, with hot flashes, night sweats, headaches, sleep disruptions, and reduced sexual drive.

But it's not just the effects of fertility drugs that can disrupt sleep. The hyperfocus of trying to become pregnant, undergoing various tests and procedures, having sex on a timetable—all of this can produce an extraordinary amount of stress.

At lunch one day I overheard two women talking about trying in vitro fertilization. Each one told a disastrous story. They reported relationship difficulties because they were "on the clock" (so to speak) to fertilize that egg when the time was right, regardless of what they were feeling. Each one felt pressure to succeed; after all, this was expensive. And the drugs made things even worse. One of the women asked, "And sleep, did you ever sleep?" They commented that it would have helped if someone had told them insomnia would be part of the deal.

I am telling you now. If you are considering in vitro fertilization, or going through it, expect poor sleep. To improve the quality of your sleep, I strongly suggest you try the worry book described in Chapter 1. Choose a time in the afternoon when you can wallow in worry and concern. Do it thoroughly and well, but do it in writing in your worry book. Remember to focus on the positive, but think clearly about the negative. That negative may be larger than life now. If you cannot get it into focus, seek professional help.

You need a firm commitment from your partner to help you through this. You'll have to have soothing support, massages, assistance with relaxation techniques, and peace. Both of you need to know that the process can cause considerable strain on the marriage, preclude a nor-

Food as a Sleep Aid

The major sleep aid in food is the amino acid tryptophan, which is converted to serotonin in nerve cells in the brain and helps modulate sleep. It takes around forty-five minutes to an hour for this conversion to take place. Milk (and dairy products), as part of its protein, contains tryptophan. So do bananas and other fruits and vegetables.

However, too much protein can be detrimental because the proteins compete to cross into the brain. It's best to limit your intake of protein to those most rich in tryptophan and avoid other proteins for a few hours before your "sleep snack." For instance, turkey and fish contain tryptophan, beef does not. Dairy products and most complex carbohydrates contain much less protein than meat or fish. Complex carbohydrates also boost levels of serotonin in the brain, which can help promote sleep. This is why we may feel sleepy after eating bread, pasta, potatoes, or cookies. So a sleep-promoting snack should include foods high in tryptophan and complex carbohydrates (which also help settle the stomach).

Avoid spicy condiments, alcohol, and citrus juices, which can irritate the esophagus, causing indigestion and acid reflux. Ditto for foods that promote stomach acid and gas, such as carbonated and caffeine-containing beverages (decaffeinated coffee can also promote stomach acid). Foods that relax the sphincter valve between the stomach and the esophagus, allowing backflow of acid from the stomach, include chocolate, peppermint, caffeinated beverages, fatty or greasy foods, fried foods, cream sauces, butter, margarine and mayonnaise, pastries, salad dressings, and whole-milk dairy products. So that evening glass of milk should be low-fat or skim if you're prone to reflux (remember, the lower the fat content, the higher the calcium).

Foods high in tryptophan include

- Milk
- Cottage cheese
- Yogurt
- Hard cheese
- Turkey
- Fish

- Bananas
- Plantains
- Dates
- Avocados
- Eggplants
- Walnuts

Your Sleep Rx for Pregnancy and Postpartum

My advice to pregnant women and new mothers is usually the same:

• First and foremost, get help! You are going to become progressively more tired and will have a heavy load to tote around. Don't make it harder on yourself.

• Take a nap if you feel like it. The National Sleep Foundation survey showed that pregnant women did make up for sleep fragmentation at night by taking naps. Find a comfortable spot for your nap. Recliners can be great, since they elevate your feet and support your back so you can breathe more easily, and they keep gastric fluids in your stomach. You can even sleep in a recliner at night.

• Putting a pillow between your knees while you lie in bed will take the strain off your back and help reduce back pain, which can cause wakefulness. Ask for a massage to ease tense muscles. Special pregnancy pillows are great, but you can use whatever you have to accomplish the same thing. You'll need those pillows especially during the third trimester, of course, when sleep can be especially difficult. The National Sleep Foundation recommends sleeping on your left side to allow the best blood flow to the uterus and kidneys.

• Avoid nighttime indigestion by eating your major meal in the middle of the day. Elevate the head of your bed four to six inches, and avoid spicy late-night snacks. Gastric reflux during sleep can cause nighttime sweats that wake you up.

• Use food as a sleep aid (see the box on page 65). During pregnancy small frequent meals can help avoid indigestion. That same strategy, eating the proper foods in the evening, can help you sleep. Dairy products will not only give you the extra calcium you need right now but also give you a dose of tryptophan that will help you sleep. Since constipation can be a problem, that nighttime snack of a high-fiber cereal and skim milk will provide you with several benefits at once. If you're taking calcium supplements, by all means save the second pill for evening. I hope you're carefully avoiding caffeine in coffee and tea, but pay extra attention to foods that can be stimulating (see the list on pages 33–34).

• You need to relax, just as any other person with a sleep problem does. Learn some relaxation techniques, like deep breathing, to help your mind and body relax (see pages 30–31). They can also help when contractions hit.

• If you're having hot flashes or night sweats postpartum, read over the tips for cooling things down on page 77. Sleep in the lightest-weight cotton gowns or pajamas you can find.

• If you find that keeping your newborn close by helps you sleep peacefully, by all means, do that. But don't feel guilty if you need to move the baby to the nursery because every little movement triggers your hormonal hyperalertness and interferes with your needed periods of sleep. This is a very individual thing.

Having a baby takes a lot out of you. The two days in the hospital after giving birth typically allowed by managed care are not adequate to regain strength. We're tired, irritable, emotional. Sleep can help.

mal sex life, and bring up financial worries. You need to be together in your goal. If your fertility clinic offers social work or psychological counseling, please take it.

No Melatonin Miracles

It was once believed that levels of melatonin decrease as we age, and that was one reason sleep became disrupted in later life. But a 1999 study reported in the *American Journal of Medicine* found that wasn't so.

In fact, a group of thirty-four healthy men and women aged sixty-five to eighty-one had melatonin levels similar to those of a control group of ninety-eight men and women eighteen to thirty years old. So, from this study, at least, there appears to be no reason to take melatonin supplements when we age.

Melatonin is sold as a supplement in health food stores, and there have been many claims over the years that it can slow the effects of aging, aid sleep, and combat jet lag. But this study seems to argue against taking extra melatonin in later life. (Another recent study found melatonin had little or no effect on jet lag.)

Melatonin is known to change circadian rhythms, or the phase in which we sleep, if it's taken at the right time. Studies examining the sedating effects of the hormone are showing mixed results. Along with its ability to substitute for the effect of light on the circadian system of the totally blind, melatonin may inhibit ovarian function (which may interfere with periods and fertility). It also contracts smooth muscle tissue, such as in artery walls, and in people with already narrowed arteries it could impair blood flow to the heart, causing angina. Women are more prone to "silent" ischemia, reduced blood flow to the heart muscle, and may not even feel chest pain or angina. So I don't recommend taking melatonin, especially if you have heart disease.

Sleep During Midlife: No Bed of Roses

I had a doctor tell me when I was thirty-five: "From here on, kid, anything goes. Your hormones will be doing crazy things for the next twenty years. So, don't think *you're* crazy. *They* are!" At the time I thought he was a little crazy himself. But now, at age sixty, I tell women of that age the same thing. First, it's probably true. Second, it allows us to stop blaming ourselves for things that are essentially out of our control (it isn't you, it's your hormones). Third, it changes treatment recommendations in some cases. And fourth, it gives you an end point, even if it is years down the road.

Perimenopause can play havoc with sleep. When estrogen begins to decline, the change may be very bothersome to women whose systems are more sensitive to the hormone (many of the same women whose sensitivities caused PMS). Surveys find that two-thirds of women complain of insomnia during the years leading up to menopause, and many researchers have documented their difficulty with falling and staying sleep, frequent awakenings, and depression.

Changes in ovarian function and reproductive hormones actually begin ten years or more (usually in your forties) before your periods stop. The unpredictable ups and downs of hormones during perimenopause upset the normal feedback loop among the ovaries, the hypothalamus, and the pituitary gland.

As our ovaries make less estrogen, our follicles become resistant to follicle-stimulating hormone (FSH). So the hypothalamus signals the pituitary to pump out more FSH in an effort to get them going again. Higher FSH is a marker of menopause, even though we may still have some monthly bleeding. Pulses of luteinizing hormone (LH) also get bigger. The effect of all this is to cause spikes in estrogen, which prompts the hypothalamus to pump out more of another hormone (gonadotropin-releasing hormone, or GnRH) to stimulate the pituitary to keep up. This hormonal roller coaster is what's believed to trigger menopausal symptoms; the hypothalamus also regulates blood pressure, body temperature, sleep and waking, appetite, sexual behavior, and mood.

A recent study at the Weill College of Medicine at Cornell University found higher LH levels in menopausal women reporting sleep disturbances and suggests that this phenomenon may be associated with hormonal changes that trigger hot flashes and night sweats. What do those symptoms do? They make us hot. What promotes sleep? Lowering the body temperature. And what's regulating this? The hypothalamic-pituitary-gonadal axis.

On the whole, perimenopausal women show more sleep disruption and mood changes than premenopausal women. Many researchers suggest a relationship between mood changes and sleep disruption. Women undergoing natural perimenopause (as opposed to surgical menopause, which occurs when the ovaries are removed during a total hysterectomy) had a 1.5 times higher risk of trouble sleeping than did younger women. In both cases stress made things worse.

Dr. Joan Shaver (who devised those Four Rs of Sleep) looked at sleep, psychological stress, and physical symptoms in perimenopausal women aged forty to fifty-nine and found that those who complained of poor sleep frequently had good sleep when measured objectively in the sleep lab. But these women also reported more stress and body symptoms, such as muscle pain, than did women with no sleep complaints. The women who did have poor sleep reported menopausal symptoms such as hot flashes. So poor sleep may be an *indirect* effect of hormonal fluctuations.

What happens when we add estrogen replacement?

Estrogen in humans enhances REM sleep, increases the time spent in REM sleep, and reduces the time it takes to get to REM sleep. Placebo-controlled studies (which tell us whether something is a real effect or just caused by people believing that a drug will work) involving pre- and postmenopausal women find that estrogen replacement helps women go to sleep faster, decreases wakefulness after falling asleep, and increases total sleep time. The more insomnia you have, the greater the benefit of hormone replacement therapy (HRT). Studies also show that women who opt for hormone replacement have more symptoms and sleep disturbances than women who don't choose HRT.

We have a lot of evidence. But we're not even close to saying we've solved the crime. Plus, there are other things going on during this transition in a woman's life that can cause stress and emotional upsets, which also disrupt sleep. Remember, the same chemical messengers that regulate mood (and are involved in depression) are involved in sleep. One of the hallmarks of depression is poor sleep.

The presence of life stresses is one of the reasons that research on sleep during midlife is so unclear. How can you separate all these influences? You probably can't.

Zapped by Hot Flashes: Should You Try Estrogen?

No doubt about it: Most women suffer from hot flashes during the perimenopausal and menopausal years, and the hot flashes interfere with sleep. At any hour of the night, you can find yourself swimming in your bed—swimming in sweat, that is.

I should tell you that the hot flash is not just a sweat flash, it is a total body and brain surge. Excitatory neurotransmitters (those brain messenger chemicals) flourish and act to alert us, wake us up as though a fire alarm rang. Many women have a hard time getting back to sleep after changing the sheets and mopping up. Once they do, another flash strikes.

A study by Drs. Kathryn Lee and Diana Taylor found that 19 percent of women as young as forty to forty-four reported awakening due to hot flashes. As women moved closer to menopause, at age forty-five to forty-nine, more than 40 percent were awakened by hot flashes. The peak age for hot flashes is fifty to fifty-four, with 43 percent reporting sleep disruptions, and the incidence started to decline as a woman moved toward her sixties.

However, there is a cure for hot flashes. Stabilizing estrogen levels with low-dose estrogen replacement, soy products, or other herbals will lessen or prevent hot flashes.

There are several forms of replacement estrogen in a variety of doses. The most commonly used form is conjugated estrogen (Premarin), derived from the urine of pregnant mares. There are other forms of estrogens (Estrace, Ortho-Est, Ogen), including a new conjugated version (Cenestin) derived from soy, and plant estrogens (Estratab, Menest). If you have a uterus, you'll need to take a synthetic progestin or a natural progesterone; talk to your doctor about the timing and the dose. Some women also find taking small doses of testosterone helps libido. Really, each woman needs an individualized regimen. An estrogen that works for one woman may not work as well (or at all) for another; the same goes for dose levels. It's something you have to work out by trial and error with your physician. I don't think anyone could say that one form of estrogen aids sleep better than another; it's the degree of symptom relief you achieve that's important.

Whether to take postmenopausal hormones is a major decision best made with advice from your physician. Consider it well, since there are so many benefits. For one thing, estrogen helps prevent bone loss and fractures caused by osteoporosis. Studies show that taking the equivalent of 0.625 milligram a day of conjugated estrogen can decrease the risk of osteoporosis and fractures by 30 to 60 percent; estrogen patches can also help prevent bone loss. (In women with already thinning bones, adding bone-building drugs to estrogen can stem the tide.)

A number of major studies show that estrogen may help decrease the risk of developing cardiovascular disease and stroke by 25 to 50 percent. This is partly because of estrogen's favorable effects on cholesterol (raising the "good" high-density lipoprotein cholesterol, HDL, and lowering the "bad" low-density lipoprotein, LDL). Estrogen helps keep blood vessels flexible, preventing age-related rises in blood pressure, and allows fewer cholesterol-laden plaques to clog arteries.

Some studies suggest that estrogen may also help prevent Alzheimer's disease and improve mood and cognitive functioning. Others suggest that estrogen may also help prevent colon cancer. Estrogen replacement can help prevent atrophy of vaginal tissues.

But estrogen is not without risks. More than fifty studies of hormone replacement and breast cancer have shown an increased risk of breast cancer, especially with long-term use of estrogen (over ten years). However, the risk is slight, around 10 percent, and short-term use (less than five years) for menopausal symptoms is not associated with an increased risk of breast cancer. Taking "unopposed" estrogen (that is, without progesterone) can lead to an overgrowth of cells in the uterine lining and an eight times greater risk of endometrial cancer. So women with an intact uterus must take progesterone to protect the uterus. (New studies also show a very slight risk with progesterone.) Recent research also suggests that estrogen replacement in women may carry a slightly increased risk of causing heart attacks, strokes, or blood clots during the first two years of treatment.

There are newer hormones, called selective estrogen receptor modulators, or SERMs (including tamoxifen, raloxifene, droloxifene, toremifene). These hormones seem to act as estrogens on the bones and the cardiovascular system but not in the breasts and uterus. However, raloxifene, the only available SERM currently prescribed for menopausal women, does not ease hot flashes; in fact, it may often make them worse. It's prescribed to prevent osteoporosis. Right now, these are products to consider after your hot flashes have subsided.

One word of advice: If you decide to try hormone replacement and still have frustrating symptoms—including sleep loss—don't give up. There are many new products on the market, and one may be perfect for you.

Dousing Hot Flashes

Other remedies can help douse those sleep-robbing hot flashes.

Soy Protein: Soy contains plant estrogens, or phytoestrogens, called isoflavones, which seem to have some of the same effects as replacement estrogen but, because they are much less potent, may carry fewer risks. Some research suggests that eating 20 to 50 grams of soy protein a day may lessen the frequency and intensity of hot flashes. One recent study at the Bowman Gray School of Medicine in Winston-Salem, North Carolina, found that women who drank an 8-ounce soy beverage each day had fewer night sweats and hot flashes than women who drank an identically flavored carbohydrate beverage. (Try the recipe for a soy smoothie on page 40.)

There are many ways you can incorporate soy into your diet: take soy supplements, drink soy milk (or milk shakes made with soy protein powder), use soy flour for baking, eat soybeans (or dry-roasted as soy nuts), and incorporate soy meat substitutes or tofu into various recipes. Tofu comes in extrafirm, firm, soft, and silken varieties (some are made with calcium sulfate, offering a second benefit). Silken tofu has a custardy consistency and is ideal for puddings and sauces (it's also lower in fat). One to two servings a day of soy may help ease your menopausal symptoms (especially hot flashes). A single serving amounts to 1 cup of soy milk, two soy hot dogs, a third of a cup of dry-roasted soy nuts, or a soyburger. Not everyone likes the taste of tofu, which needs lots of seasonings to overcome its soy flavor. A trove of tasty tofu and soy recipes can be found in *Estrogen: The Natural Way,* by Nina Shandler (Villard, 1997), a cookbook aimed at midlife women. You can also get isoflavones from lentils, chickpeas, and beans.

Another plant estrogen is flaxseed. It contains a potent phytoestrogen called lignan, and some studies suggest it can also ease hot flashes (but there's much less research on flaxseed than on soy). Flaxseed also contains important vitamins and minerals, including potassium, iron, and B vitamins, plus it's a soluble fiber (like oatmeal) and can be a great source of fiber in your diet. (Flaxseed is also incorporated into many recipes in Shandler's book.)

Herbs: Many herbs, including fennel, dong quai (angelica root), red clover, and black cohosh *(Cimicifuga racemosa),* are also phytoestrogens. Black cohosh contains substances that act similarly to estrogens; dong quai supposedly helps the body use available estrogen made by fatty tissue. Studies suggest both can help hot flashes, vaginal dryness, and mood disturbances (although their safety is still being tested). Black cohosh is also sold as tinctures, syrup, or dried root. (The generally accepted dose is 40 grams a day in tablets, tinctures, or tea.) Dong quai is often sold as a liquid or as cured root. Red clover is a source of potent isoflavones, which are chemically similar to estrogen.

There are herbal supplements that may help ease hot flashes and other menopausal symptoms. Remifemin, black cohosh in tablets (20 milligrams standardized dose each), has been clinically tested in Europe and in the United States. Another clinically tested herbal menopausal supplement is Promensil, made from red clover, a potent source of estrogenic isoflavones (each tablet contains 40 milligrams of various isoflavones). Studies of Promensil found a more than 50 percent reduction in hot flashes in women taking the supplement, without overgrowth of the uterine lining.

Some women swear by ginseng to curb hot flashes. The root of the ginseng plant is a potent phytoestrogen used in Eastern medicine in tea and other preparations to relieve hot flashes, aches, and pains, as well as to boost energy and (allegedly) sex drive. However, ginseng also has estrogenic effects in the body. Some studies suggest that it may stimulate overgrowth of the endometrial lining, and large amounts can cause high blood pressure, gastrointestinal problems, and insomnia.

How Safe Are Herbs?

Like many medically oriented clinicians, I have little firsthand knowledge of herbal products other than what I have gleaned from reading and talking to my colleagues. Therefore, as you read this, remember that I too am still learning.

If you're thinking about using herbal products, it's important to note that even though all these products are considered "natural," they also need to be regarded as drugs. Herbs change brain chemicals, and they may well interfere with other medications you're on or other aspects of your body functions. So be alert to the fact that they can cause side effects, some quite serious.

In general, herbs are thought to offer more gentle effects than other pharmaceuticals with, we hope, fewer side effects. But it's also important to understand that herbs have multiple effects, and may produce more than one response. In general, herbalists like to think of them as offering a sort of a tonic effect, establishing a homeostasis or balance in the body.

However, many herbs haven't been thoroughly tested in placebo-controlled clinical trials in this country. Some, such as St. John's wort, have been extensively tested in Europe and are now being studied here. But we don't yet know the optimal dose for many preparations. And it's really hard to determine the actual potency of herbals you're buying.

Legally, herbs are dietary supplements, *not* drugs, so manufacturers aren't allowed to claim that they prevent or treat disease. Food and Drug Administration regulations that went into effect in 1999 require labels on herbal products and supplements to list the concentration or percentage of active ingredients and side effects. It's always wise to buy a product with one herb as opposed to several, since concentrations of the desired herb may be lower and other ingredients may cause unwanted side effects.

Ads for brand-name herbs and supplements promise more "complete" and reliable "nondrug" remedies, but much of this is hype. Herbs do act as drugs, but there's *no* potency guarantee for herbs as there is for drugs. When a drug says "USP" on the label, that means the U.S. Pharmacopeial Convention has stipulated that it must contain a specified percentage of the active ingredient. If it doesn't meet those specifications, it's subpotent and cannot be sold as a drug, or it can't carry the label USP. With a botanical that's non-USP, there's no guarantee the active ingredient is present in any meaningful concentration. Brand names may have an advantage, however, in assuring you of uniformity from dose to dose. You don't have any assurance that it's the *right* dose. But you can largely trust the manufacturers to maintain more or less the *same* dose from bottle to bottle.

Because as yet there's no agreement on formulations, I can't recommend specific doses of herbs. What I *do* recommend is that you read labels carefully. Just as with medications, you can take too much of an herb. Discuss herbs and supplements with your doctor before you take them, and report any difficulties immediately. Likewise, tell alternative practitioners about any over-the-counter or prescription medicines you're taking.

I'd do some homework and check products out thoroughly before buying. A good place to start would be at reputable sites on the World Wide Web. Check out the USP Web site at www.usp.org, the FDA's Web site at www.fda.gov, and the National Institutes of Health, www.nal.usda.gov/fnic/IBIDS. Some manufacturers, among them the makers of Remifemin and Promensil, have done extensive research on their products and provide information on their Web sites.

Your local library may also have copies of the *Physicians' Desk Reference for Herbal Medicines* (Medical Economics Publishing, 1998). Germany's Commission E, the equivalent of our FDA, has issued recommendations for herbal products, which are sold as drugs in Germany. Detailed guidelines can be found in *The Complete German Commission E Monographs: Therapeutic Guide to Herbal Medicines,* first edition (Blumenthal, American Botanical Council, 1998), also in many libraries. Other good books include *Rational Phytotherapy,* by Shultz, Hantzel, and Tyler (Purdue University, School of Pharmacy and Pharmaceutical Science). Varo Tyler is a well-respected authority on herbals.

Please *do* check with your doctor before using *any* herbal product! Do *not* use phytoestrogens if you're taking hormone replacement therapy. (For more information about herbs and how to use them, see the box on pages 78–80.)

There are a number of other remedies for hot flashes recommended by menopause experts. Among them are the following:

VITAMIN E is said to help douse flashes. There haven't been any studies to back up that claim, but many women swear by it. The recommended dose ranges from 400 to 600 international units twice a day. Remember, vitamins are powerful drugs and those, like vitamin E, that are fat-soluble can accumulate in the body and be toxic in high doses. So don't overdo it and consult your physician beforehand.

If you can't or won't take estrogen replacement and you have frequent, severe hot flashes, consider the following in consultation with your doctor.

CLONIDINE (CATAPRES) is a high blood pressure medication that relaxes blood vessels. Studies show it can reduce hot flashes by 20 to 45 percent, though not as effectively as estrogen. In higher doses clonidine can cause dry mouth, insomnia, and faintness. This drug is available as a skin patch that's worn on the shoulder and replaced once a week.

METHYLDOPA (ALDOMET) is another antihypertensive, which may cut down on hot flashes by as much as 30 percent. Side effects include nausea, dizziness, and fatigue.

BELLERGAL is a tranquilizer, a combination of belladonna, ergotamine, and phenobarbital, which may help with hot flashes, sleep problems, irritability, mood swings, and headaches.

As a sleep specialist, I can only tell you what has been helpful for a particular sleep problem. We don't usually prescribe medications for menopausal symptoms. These are drugs best taken under the direction of your gynecologic physician. As for me, before I started estrogen, my hot flashes were so severe that I stood out on my deck in the snow in my bare feet fanning myself; my family thought I'd lost my mind, but it sure cooled me down. I don't recommend that approach. Here are some better ways of coping with hot flashes and night sweats:

• Keep your bedroom cool. An overly warm bedroom can make hot flashes feel even worse. (If your partner is cold, try one of those dual-control electric blankets.)

• Wear cotton nightgowns or pajamas to bed. Cotton absorbs moisture and allows body heat to escape. Cotton sheets are also cooler than blends.

You may want to keep an extra nightgown or pair of pajamas by the

Herbal Remedies

Herbal Product	Possible Action	Formulation
HERBS TO COMBAT PMS SYMPTOMS		
Black cohosh root	Estrogenlike activity	Capsule, tablet
Bugleweed (breast pain)	Mild antigonadotropic	Tea, extract
Chaste tree fruit	Anti-inflammatory	Extract
Dandelion	Mild diuretic	Dried leaves for tea
Ginseng root (fatigue)	Stimulant, plant estrogen	Bulk herb, dried root for tea, capsule
Kava kava	Eases stress, anxiety	Tincture, extract, capsule, tablet
Evening primrose oil	Essential fatty acids reduce inflammation	Capsule
St. John's wort	Boosts serotonin, eases depression	Hypericum extract, capsule
Valerian root	Sedative properties	Tincture, extract, capsule, tea
Yarrow (pelvic cramps)	Anti-inflammatory, pain reliever	Dried herb or tea
HERBS TO COMBAT BLOATING, ABDOMINAL FULLNESS		
Angelica root	Antispasmodic aids mild intestinal spasms, flatulence, fullness	Bulk herb
Chamomile	Antispasmodic for gastrointestinal complaints	Bulk herb, flowers for tea
Caraway seed and oil	Mild antispasmodic, combats flatulence	Oil, dried seeds for infusion**
Dandelion herb	Mild diuretic	Tincture, tea, dried or fresh leaves
Fennel seed and oil	Muscle relaxant, antispasmodic	Tincture, dry bulk ground seeds
Gentian root	Digestive aid	Dried root (for tea), tincture
Peppermint leaves	Antispasmodic of digestive tract	Tea, tincture, fresh or dried

Herbal Product	Possible Action	Formulation
HERBS TO EASE MENSTRUAL CRAMPS		
Black cohosh root	Estrogenlike action	Capsule, tablet
Potentilla	Tannins ease mild menstrual cramps	Powdered, cut herbs for infusion**
Primrose oil	Essential fatty acids reduce inflammation	Capsule, oil
HERBS TO EASE MENOPAUSAL SYMPTOMS		
Black cohosh root (Remifemin, MenoBalance)	Estrogenlike activity	Tablet, capsule
Red clover (Promensil)	Plant estrogen	Tablet
Ginseng*	Stimulant	Tea, dried root
Kava kava	Reduces anxiety, stress	Tincture, extract, capsule, tablet
Licorice root*	Anti-inflammatory	Tea or extract
Motherwort herb (rapid heartbeat)	Alkaloids act on cardiac function	Powder, herbs for infusion**
St. John's wort	Increases serotonin, eases depression	Hypericum extract, capsule
Indian snakeroot (rapid heartbeat)	Mild alpha and beta blocker action	Powder, capsule
Valerian root	Sedative properties	Tincture, extract, capsule, tea
HERBS TO HELP INSOMNIA		
Hops	Essential oils ease mood, anxiety	Powder or dry extract, liquid
Lavender flower	Essential oils ease insomnia, restlessness	Extract, oil, herbs for tea
Lemon balm	Sedative, eases gastrointestinal complaints	Dried/ground herb, extract, tea
Passionflower	Alkaloid compound eases nervousness, restlessness	Herb for tea
Valerian root	Sedative	Tincture, extract, capsule, tea

Herbal Product	Possible Action	Formulation
HERBS TO EASE LEG CRAMPS		
Butcher's broom	Eases vein swelling, leg pain, heaviness	Extract
Horse chestnut seed (Venastat)	Eases vein and leg swelling, leg pain	Tincture, capsule
Sweet clover	Eases vein and leg swelling, night cramps	Herb for infusion,** liquid

*Caution: Ginseng and licorice root can raise blood pressure.
**For information on infusions see page 103.

Sources: *Physicians' Desk Reference for Herbal Medicines* (Medical Economics Publishing, 1998); *The Complete German Commission E Monographs: Therapeutic Guide to Herbal Medicines,* 1st ed. (Blumenthal, American Botanical Council, 1998).

bed, along with some moist facial towelettes. That way you don't have to feel your way to the dresser in the dark.

• Avoid those sleep disrupters caffeine and alcohol. Both can trigger hot flashes.

• Find ways to reduce stress in your life (stress can be a hot flash trigger). Relaxation exercises can help. So can regular exercise; it may increase levels of the body's feel-good hormones called endorphins, which may also help lessen hot flashes. See suggestions for relaxation exercises on pages 30–31.

Your Sleep Rx for Midlife

I'm always happy to see women come to the Sleep Disorders Center when they start having menopausal symptoms, so I can short-circuit any long-term problems.

This is the time to rehearse or establish those really good sleep habits discussed in Chapter 1, because there is the real likelihood that things will get worse before they get better. Clearly, sleep is worse in the years leading up to and during menopause. Peri-menopausal women have much more sleep fragmentation than premenopausal women. This is a time when the practice of good sleep hygiene is very helpful. And the hot flashes *will* pass.

Women with depression, especially those who suffer PMS, may experience many more symptoms (and that includes sleep disruptions) at menopause. We know that midlife women have the highest risk of mood disorders.

I am very much in favor of psychiatric involvement at this time. You may not need medications, but psychotherapy could forestall symptoms of depression in the same way that good sleep hygiene prevents insomnia. A few preventive strikes may be in order.

Here are some other tips for maximizing sleep at midlife.

• I recommend learning ways to reduce stress through relaxation exercises, biofeedback, acupuncture, yoga, or tai chi (don't forget Kegel exercises to strengthen the pelvic floor and reduce urinary incontinence; see page 111).

• Many gynecologists advocate taking 200 milligrams of timed-release vitamin B_6 (pyridoxine) for women taking hormones of any kind to reduce side effects and help mood.

• Consider soy and herbs. Evening primrose oil and teas made with chamomile and red raspberry leaves are also said to relieve menopausal symptoms. Many herbs can be steeped as teas, and some taste quite pleasant. But remember the cautions I listed in the chart on pages 78–80. Ask your doctor about soy or herbal menopausal supplements.

• Try taking extra calcium and magnesium. Calcium may help reduce irritability, insomnia, and headaches during menopause. Magnesium helps balance hormones and can also ease some vasomotor symptoms of menopause, like heart palpitations.

• Gastric reflux may be to blame for some nighttime sweats. In gastric reflux, stomach acid backs up into the esophagus and stimulates the vagus nerve, setting off vascular symptoms and cough. A simple test is to try one of the acid blocker medications (such as Tagamet or Pepcid) and see if your sweats disappear. However, check with your physician first. You can sleep on extra pillows (although sometimes elevating just the head can aggravate things) or elevate the entire head of the bed with wood or cinder blocks placed under the legs, using gravity to help keep stomach acid where it belongs.

• If you are waking up to go to the bathroom several times a night, you may have an overactive bladder (see page 110). Medication can help, but be aware that there are side effects, such as dry mouth, that may compound hormonal changes (which also cause drying of tissues). If the problem is not overactive bladder, you might try behavioral modification. This includes reducing liquids in the evening and bladder retraining.

• If you take progesterone and estrogen in separate pills for hormone replacement, take your progesterone after dinner. As I mentioned, progesterone can have sleep-inducing effects. There's no guarantee it will help you sleep better, but it's worth a try.

Women's Ages and Stages of Sleep

Navigating Your Nights

Too many of us accept sleep problems as part of our lives. We see our male partners sacked out in front of the TV while we're sorting the socks, or find ourselves heating a cup of milk in the wee hours of the morning while everyone else is blissfully asleep. Somehow, we figure, men must simply sleep better. At least they seem to sleep more and get to sleep more easily. We manage with less sack time, right? Maybe we women just need less sleep.

Not true.

As I've discussed, there are differences in men's and women's sleep patterns, some of which have to do with hormones and gender. But many of the problems women face with sleep have to do with life stages and situations.

Sleep problems among women typically emerge during the child-bearing years, when many of us are trying to juggle work and home life, tending to careers, marriages, and children. Some of us must work the night shift. Most of us have worked "the second shift," following our day job with child care. But there are just so many hours in the day, and something's got to give. That something is usually sleep.

Being pregnant and caring for an infant have profound impacts on our sleep. In addition to the hormonal aspects of pregnancy and child-birth, there are the physical stresses of pregnancy and the demands of taking care of a newborn who needs to be fed on a schedule (day and night). In our striving to do our best as parents, sleep often gets put on the back burner. Postpartum depression or anxiety may be overlooked as a cause of sleep problems because we expect disrupted sleep at this time of life.

Midlife may bring added responsibilities, with many of us caring for aging parents and children at the same time. When we hit perimenopause, symptoms such as hot flashes and perhaps depression can also take their toll. If you're unhappy about approaching midlife, or if life changes are stressing you, you may feel the impact at night.

Older age can bring changes in sleep patterns; physical ailments like arthritis or overactive bladder can keep us awake. Some older women may have health problems that require relocation to a nursing home, and that brings its own set of sleep disrupters.

Understanding the life stage you're in is important to getting a good night's sleep.

On the Yawn Patrol

The National Sleep Foundation's 2000 Omnibus Sleep in America Poll found that 43 percent of the people surveyed complained of excessive daytime sleepiness. Many had medically significant sleepiness, based on the Epworth Sleepiness Scale (see page 15). Over a third of the people surveyed said that sleepiness interfered with their daytime activities. Over half said it interfered with their driving, and many of these were women!

Amazingly, many people who report daytime sleepiness think that it's not a serious problem! Sleep ranked third among health concerns.

And it's not just Americans who are sleepy. A Canadian study of almost three thousand young adults showed that two-thirds reported some complaints about sleep. Furthermore, women aged seventeen to thirty had more nightmares, delayed sleep onset, and more frequent arousal than did men the same age. (It seems more of the younger men took naps.)

I have seen too many women trying to "do it all," maintain careers while shouldering too many responsibilities at home. We all have multiple roles we must play, and there's often no supporting cast (74 percent of single parents are women).

The Art of Napping

Naps are best when kept short (less than thirty minutes, certainly not more than forty). The shorter the nap, the less likely you will fall into a nighttime pattern of sleep and wake up groggy. Find a comfortable, quiet place (turn off the ringer on your desk phone, or have your calls routed to voice mail). Ideally you want to lie down, or lie back on the couch with your feet on an ottoman. But you can also put your head in your arms at your desk or the kitchen table. (In a vehicle, I pull over and use a neck collar to keep my head from rolling.) Close your eyes, focus on your breathing, and all of a sudden you'll be drifting off. It's as simple as that. Stretch after your nap to work out any muscle kinks.

What's the best time for a workday nap? Sometime between 2:00 and 4:00 P.M., when there's a natural dip in alertness. Can't afford a couch in your office? Try the floor with an exercise mat (but warn your co-workers). Don't have an office? Put your head in your arms or sit back in your chair with a neck pillow to support your head. Or you might make "time out" arrangements at your company's health office.

Think you'll need a note for clearance? Ask your physician. Most workplaces would substitute a nap break for a coffee break, especially if doing so increased employee effectiveness. You'll be a trendsetter. (If your work is at home, you've got on-site napping facilities.)

According to a 1998 report by the Families and Work Institute, although men appear to be pitching in more these days, women spend almost three hours doing chores on workdays and almost six hours on nonworkdays (almost an hour a day more than their male partners). Women spend more than three hours daily caring for and doing things with their children during the workweek (compared with two and a third hours for men), and more than eight hours daily on weekends (versus not quite six and a half hours for the men). Of course there's always overlap; we can be cooking dinner and supervising homework at the same time. This second shift comes on top of a workweek that averages between forty and forty-six hours for women (men spent longer hours at work). Child rearing itself can cause sleep disturbances. When

Your Second Shift Sleep Rx

How you organize your day can affect how well you'll sleep at night.

For working women, whether that work is in the home or at an office, the biggest need is to set priorities, and make yourself one of them.

Frazzled at mealtimes? Who decreed that gourmet meals are necessary every night? Okay, no one wants to live on frozen entrées or takeout. So plan a cooking marathon one weekend a month; prepare big batches of chili, lasagna, whatever favorite dishes can be made in bulk and frozen.

Involve the entire family. Shop together and consult about nutrition. Make joint decisions about menus and meal preparation. Even toddlers can toss salads, carry food, wash potatoes. Children love to cook, and they are more likely to eat what they've prepared themselves. When you arrive home from work, you (or, if you're lucky, someone else) will pop the food in the oven or microwave while you take a shower to revive.

Many working women find they experience a midafternoon "slump" when they're kind of drowsy and crave a cup of coffee and something sweet to pick them up. Others are hit by a slump in the early evening, when confronting dinner, homework, or housework after a hard day's work.

You're better off with a fifteen-minute nap at your desk than trying to get a few winks on the couch at home before tackling your evening. Napping in the early evening will disrupt your sleep patterns (see the box on page 85). A healthy midafternoon snack like fruit is better than starchy sweets, which can make you more drowsy. Use coffee wisely. The caffeine in your afternoon coffee will take fifteen to thirty minutes to start to perk you up, and it may stay in your system as long as seven hours. If you're sensitive to caffeine, have decaf. Or drink your coffee with lunch to keep you more alert in the afternoon but not interfere with sleep at night.

While I don't advise an evening nap, there's nothing wrong with crawling into bed with the kids and reading or watching a video. At least you're together and your feet are up! Some nights, even a picnic in bed is fun (if you watch the crumbs). If you find yourself dozing off, take turns with story-time duty so you can kick off your shoes and relax.

According to the National Sleep Foundation, 38 percent of adults take at least one nap during the workday (averaging around an hour). But even shorter naps are good. Several years ago I surveyed commuters on the Long Island Rail Road, the country's largest suburban commuter rail line. Many more women than men napped on the trip into the city and out at night. That surprised me because I had assumed that personal safety was an issue, but I think that concern gets overpowered by sleepiness. That short nap can be refreshing and, in my study, appeared to extend people's shortened nighttime sleep. According to the Families and Work Institute, the average commute is about forty-seven minutes, plenty of time for a brief nap. But, again, if you find the nap on the commute home is making it harder for you to fall asleep at bedtime, do some relaxing reading instead.

About one in six adults say their employers allow them to nap at work. I recently read in the newspaper that some employers are building nap time into the workday (some are actually building napping rooms!). Right now, it's mostly companies where workers have high-stress or high-responsibility jobs, such as railway engineers or airline pilots. You don't want a sleepy person at the throttle of a high-speed locomotive or jet plane. Even the U.S. Army has gotten into the act, convinced by sleep research showing that naps can help people perform better.

By the way, showers are useful as temporary wake-me-ups and nice separations between the workday and home. This is a habit I learned in nursing school. We were never allowed to carry hospital germs to our beds. Showers were mandatory. So, anytime I return from work or someplace where I've gotten a dose of germs, I shower and start over.

Of course, paid help is wonderful. But most of us can't afford a cook, a housekeeper, and someone to run errands for us. So use the help that's available: your partner and kids. Even toddlers can sort colors in a washload, find their clothes, and fold (this is a great way to learn counting and colors). Put on a tape or CD and sing while you sort. So maybe the shirts won't be folded perfectly, but, hey, what's really important here? Isn't it better to share time with the kids and lighten your load? Divvy up the errands and chores, making a jobs list if you need to. Encourage your kids to pack their own lunches. Get them into the habit of laying out their clothes and getting backpacks ready to go the night before so you're not chasing down socks or homework at dawn. Have a variety of breakfasts (cereal, toaster waffles) on hand that kids can fix for themselves so you can catch a few more minutes of sleep in the morning. When people know what's expected of them, they rise to the occasion (yes, even teens!).

You may also find that exchanging chores and baby-sitting with a neighbor or friend can be a lifesaver. Grocery buying, meal cooking, and baby-sitting can be cooperative efforts. Everybody contributes something, taking turns. Everyone benefits.

Many working women find themselves beset by anxiety about what they're *not* doing. When they're at work they worry about the kids and household matters; when they're home they worry about work. Here's where your worry book (see page 27) can help you put aside those thoughts that may trouble your sleep (and your waking hours). You may need to set aside time to talk to your partner (or your boss) about things that are worrying you. The problems that loom large at night often turn out to be small and solvable when tackled by daylight.

Finally, make sleep a priority. It is just as important to your

health as a proper diet and vitamins. But you must *make time* for
it. Let something else go. If you get any flak, tell 'em I said so! I
know from personal experience that sleep matters, and you can be
much more efficient with a good night's sleep. You'll be surprised
how easily the day goes if you think clearly and feel bright. And the
bonus is you're teaching family members that sleep is important, too.

you have young children you're always "on call," and many women
accept disrupted sleep as part and parcel of parenting. Next stop:
burnout.

All too often, women feel they don't have any choice about juggling
too many roles, and that adds another stressor that robs us of sleep. A
good example is a couple I'll call Denise and Dennis. Denise is a thirty-
six-year-old married mother of a two-year-old. She has difficulty staying
asleep and complains of waking up listless. She works in her husband's
software and computer store two to three days a week, when she can get
a relative to baby-sit. The shop is busy, but there's no money to hire
workers. Denise would rather be working at her own career in advertis-
ing, but she feels obligated to help her husband.

She leaves the shop early on her workdays so she can spend time
with her son, give him dinner, and put him to bed at 7:00 P.M. But
Dennis doesn't get home until after midnight most nights. He's attending graduate school, hoping a business degree will help him succeed.

Of course, Denise wants to spend time with her husband, and she
attempts to wait up for him so they can talk or eat together. Frequently,
however, she finds that after doing the laundry and other chores in the
evening, she falls asleep before Dennis comes home and then has difficulty getting back to sleep before 3:00 A.M. Lately, even if she doesn't
plan to wait up, she finds herself awakening between 1:00 and 3:00 A.M.,
and has a hard time getting back to sleep. Not surprisingly, it's difficult
for her to wake up in the morning, and by the time she gets up, Dennis
has already gone to the store. Their weekends are full: the shop is open

When You're Working the Night Shift

Many women work in service industries such as health care that are active over twenty-four hours. If you're like most shift workers, you work nights, then immediately shift back to a day schedule when you're off. Unfortunately, your biological clock never knows where you are, and you're continually uncomfortable (research shows sleep is not as good during the day). Women working the night shift can also experience menstrual irregularities and infertility.

Of course, some people thrive on shift work. If you're a night person who loves working late at night, you could be the happiest and healthiest of workers because your biological clock is in sync with your chosen activity. But most shift workers find themselves chronically sleep-deprived, never quite catching up.

However, there are steps you can take to make your life easier:

• Stay as much on the night shift as possible.

• If you must rotate shifts, try to go with the clock, from days to evenings to nights.

• Find an area where you can get increased lighting at night. Usually the lights are dim indoors. If possible, increase the brightness, sound, and activity to mimic day. (This is also helpful for people who work in windowless offices, who may not get enough light during the day.)

• If you work an overnight shift, wear sunglasses on the way home to avoid light.

• Some people find it hard to sleep in the morning, when alertness is naturally increased. The best time to sleep is after lunch, to take advantage of that natural energy dip (assuming your biological clock hasn't shifted). However, this can be difficult if you have school-age children. If possible, try to arrange for child care from after school until dinnertime so you can sleep.

• After dinner try to catch a nap to reduce your sleep debt and to increase alertness on the job.

• Need a little extra help? The newest sleep medication, zaleplon (Sonata), may be just the thing to help start that afternoon nap. It's short-acting and will not interfere with your performance at work later on. If you need to be extra-alert, a medication used to help people with narcolepsy, modafinil (Provigil), can help you. It's not an amphetaminelike drug that will speed you up, and it's not addictive. Talk to your doctor about these medications.

• Consider light therapy to help reset your biological clock. The consistent use of light immediately upon awakening will reset your clock in a matter of days depending on how different the wake time is from your usual. You should soon find it easier to sleep and wake at the necessary time, although once you stop using the light you will probably shift back. (For more details on light therapy, see page 161.)

on Saturday, and Sunday is taken up with housework, grocery shopping, and other errands. Denise had little free time and felt trapped.

She finally came to see me because of constant fatigue and poor sleep; she worries that she cannot keep up this pace. She's also concerned about the state of her marriage but feels she cannot alter or improve her situation. These feelings seem more overwhelming during the week before her period (yes, depression can be a symptom of PMS!). As extreme as this situation may appear, it's illustrative of a common female dilemma: too many stressors, too many responsibilities, and no way to eliminate any of them.

Denise's sleep complaint was actually the easiest thing to fix. But first she needed to organize home and business tasks with Dennis's help, to give herself some breathing room. Dennis agreed to cut back on his class load to have dinner at home with his family most nights, and he hired a part-time employee to work in the store one day a week and Saturdays. They divvied up the housework, and built in a regular "date" once a week, even if it was just taking a walk together.

To relieve Denise's insomnia, we made the following plan: Since Dennis was home most nights for dinner, Denise didn't feel as obliged to stay up late to spend time with him. I had her choose a regular bedtime and wake time. Initially, she began with a consistent wake time of 6:00 A.M., staying up late to condense her hours of sleep. As is the case for most patients, when the push and concern about sleep were over, she relaxed and found it easier to drift off at that late time. Evening naps were forbidden, so Denise busied herself with relaxing activities like sewing or reading. Within one month she had consolidated her sleep so she could go to sleep by 10:00 P.M. and stay asleep until 6:00 A.M. She also kept to the other rules of good sleep hygiene. Dennis found his sleep was helped, too. And both of them felt they had a better time in the morning, now that they could all have breakfast together.

Gaining a sense of control over her sleep, and making a plan to destress her waking hours, relieved her tension, even before Denise's sleep problems were solved. She's considering seeing a therapist to deal with her feelings of depression.

These may seem like simple steps, but they can be difficult for most women to achieve without a concerted effort. And that effort should involve your partner and children.

Sleeping Like a Baby?

Wouldn't we all like to sleep like babies again?

Female sleep differences seem to start in infancy. Girls tend to have more slow-wave sleep than boys as they grow. Around the age of thirteen to fifteen, girls begin to spend less time in bed and have shorter sleep than boys. Around age sixteen they decrease the proportion of REM sleep as well. Adolescent girls tend to have much less active dreams with much less sexual content than adolescent boys.

Even though teenage girls may have more slow-wave sleep than boys, they may also be more prone to social pressures to shortcut sleep. With the onset of menses, they must also cope with the unpredictability, cramping, and intermittent PMS of their periods. Their rapidly changing bodies cause concerns and stress. We know how much hormonal changes can affect our sleep. (Teens also have specific sleep issues, which we will discuss in Chapter 8.)

But it's during a woman's childbearing years that many sleep problems crop up. Some are caused by hormones during and after pregnancy, but other sleep problems can be caused by the demands of parenting.

The Birth of Sleep Deprivation

No one expects to sleep well during the nights spent in the hospital after giving birth: Noise, doctors and nursing staff bustling in the rooms and hallways at all hours, bright lights, the baby rooming in, and roommates (if you have a semiprivate room) all conspire to disrupt sleep no matter how tired you may be after labor and delivery.

Dr. Kathryn Lee, a nurse-researcher in San Francisco, notes that new mothers get about the same amount of sleep during the postnatal period as they did during the last trimester (okay, so it's not enough!). Dr. Lee found that after delivery women had no difficulty falling asleep, but they did have difficulty maintaining sleep (perhaps that's the one time we do fall asleep as quickly as babies!). New mothers reported more daytime fatigue and low energy, reminiscent of sleep deprivation. However, Dr. Lee found that they were experiencing not true sleep deprivation, but the effects of sleep fragmentation—grabbing sleep a few hours at a time instead of in one long rest—because of the demands of caring for a newborn. What's going on is an increase in what we call WASO (Wake After Sleep Onset) episodes, and a significant decrease in deep sleep (stages 3–4); our normal sleep patterns are interrupted by the need to feed and change the newborn.

Caring for an infant is a round-the-clock job, not unlike the situation faced by medical students, doctors, and emergency medical technicians. According to researchers at the Sleep Disorders and Research Center at the Henry Ford Hospital in Detroit, these workers may lose an hour and a half of sleep when on call, regardless of whether their pagers go off. Similarly, being "on call" as a new mother can disrupt sleep even when the baby sleeps through the night.

If you have a premature baby, you may be especially sleep-deprived, because preemies have to be fed more often than full-term babies. In this situation, I find catnaps very useful. Try to find a way to get an extra fifteen minutes of sleep a night. Even that little bit can help, and it sets an awareness that you should be thinking about increasing sleep as soon as possible rather than filling that time with yet another chore. Twins can be particularly stressful, until you get them on a synchronized sleep and feeding schedule (see pages 202–03). Stress and sleep loss are major cul-

---

That Other "Biological Clock"

Some of you may have been hearing your reproductive biological clock ticking lately. That ticking may be louder and more urgent. Is it time to have a baby? Perhaps you're losing sleep over it. Women today spend a lot of time wondering, Should I or shouldn't I? If so, when? Frequently, the decision-making process is stressful, depressing, or stimulating. All of these moods can affect one's ability to sleep.

From a sleep clinician's perspective, women's sleep troubles during these years frequently revolve around childbearing issues. I would guess that about a third of my thirty-something insomniac patients are worried about this issue and losing sleep over it. Some worry for good reason. Often their husbands won't commit to having children, or have no sense of urgency (after all, they keep making more sperm). We have only so many eggs, time doesn't stop for our ovaries while we're deciding, and careers cannot always be put on hold until a partner is ready. My advice: Communicate your concerns clearly to your partner when both of you are awake, alert, and able to discuss things clearly. Also, as I mentioned in Chapter 2, remember that fertility drugs can affect your ability to sleep.

---

prits in the depressed mood and memory loss experienced by many new mothers.

Is It the "Baby Blues" or Depression?

We should be clear that the "baby blues" are not the same as post-partum depression. More than half of all new mothers will have a brief bout with the "baby blues" three to five days after delivery. You'll experience fluctuating moods: One minute you're thrilled with this new person in your life, the next you're in tears because of spilled formula, and swamped by a sense of inadequacy. You may feel overwhelmed, but you're not experiencing the deep hopelessness typical of major depression. Your mood should improve in a week or so.

Contrast this with the experience of between 10 and 15 percent of women, who have postpartum major depression (PPMD). Their symp-

---

Warning Signs of Postpartum Depression

- Feelings of despondency, worthlessness, or guilt
- Lack of appetite
- Extreme sleep disturbance (sleeping too much or too little)
- Problems with concentration or memory
- Extreme fatigue and irritability
- Excessive worry about the baby's health or feeding habits
- Feelings of inadequacy, or of being a "bad" or unloving mother

---

toms of depression and extreme sleep disturbance (see the box above) can last for weeks. Be aware that PPMD may appear weeks, months, even as much as a year after giving birth. Dr. Pat Coble, a sleep researcher at Western Psychiatric Institute in Pittsburgh, finds that women who have suffered a previous depression are more at risk for postpartum major depression. If you suspect you may have PPMD— and sleep problems are a major symptom—please seek help immediately. There's effective treatment and no need for you to suffer.

Treatments include medication and psychotherapy. Recent studies indicate that newer antidepressants, such as the selective serotonin reuptake inhibitor (SSRI) fluoxetine (Prozac) and its cousins, can safely be given to nursing mothers. These medications are secreted in only minute amounts in breast milk and do not seem to affect the baby's behavior or growth. For women at risk of postpartum depression, starting antidepressants immediately after delivery and continuing for three months may help prevent a recurrence. Women who have suffered episodes of manic depression or bipolar disorder (wide swings between euphoria and deep depression) can also be helped with prophylactic regimens of lithium and other drugs.

New research also shows that the tricyclic antidepressants (TCAs) like desipramine (Norpramin) and nortriptyline (Aventyl, Pamelor), which have fewer side effects than other TCAs, and the newer SSRIs like fluoxetine, fluvoxamine (Luvox), paroxetine (Paxil), and sertraline (Zoloft), can safely be given during pregnancy, when symptoms of

The New Mom's Sleep Rx

I am frequently asked by journalists what new mothers can do to get sleep immediately after delivery. My answer is always the same: Nap. Catch some sleep when the baby does, especially if you're breast feeding. A thirty-minute nap can also help make up for sleep lost to being "on call." It fact, that's what many mothers reported doing in the National Sleep Foundation's women and sleep survey! Naps can be very useful additions to our twenty-four-hour sleep patterns if we take them regularly. Southern Hemispheric countries have regular siestas, don't they? For new moms, I advise planning a fairly regular nap time during the day, preferably in the early afternoon, when our biologic propensity to sleep is greatest. At least put your head down. Turn off the phone. Turn the baby monitor down a bit while your newborn is safe in the crib. Thirty minutes is a good amount of time to allow. That refreshes you for a couple of hours and prevents the descent into deeper sleep. If you sleep longer, you risk falling into your regular sleep rhythm of deep sleep. When you awaken, you'll be groggy, hungover, and possibly grumpy. If you are very sleep-deprived, that may even happen after a short nap. Just be aware that you may not be able to jump up and react quickly, especially at first. Try to get the baby in sync with your own nap time. If you can't get your baby on a nap schedule, put him or her in a safe crib or playpen with safe distractions (approved mobiles and toys) and rest assured that your baby will let you know if he or she really needs you.

Unfortunately, napping isn't used as a strategy as often as we'd like. There's always a load of laundry, a sink full of dishes, a pile of work on the desk. You may feel unproductive and guilty if you're not using this downtime to get something done. Everyone tells you to "sleep when the baby sleeps," but you're determined to have something more than a pile of used diapers to show for the day. Please, for the sake of your health, let it go. I've seen new mothers dig themselves into really serious sleep deficits, making their anxiety and depression much worse, when naps could have prevented such an outcome.

Employers grant maternity leave for time off from work after childbirth, but too few women give *themselves* time off. Give yourself a break. Be unproductive once (or twice) a day. Take a nap. Your body will thank you for it.

Give up some control. Ask for and accept help. Ask your partner to take over a nighttime feeding, with expressed milk or formula. Hire a baby-sitter to watch your newborn while you nap, and tell yourself this is for your health, not a luxury. In previous eras we were blessed with family living close; our own mothers and grandmothers were available for advice and help. If yours live nearby and are willing, allow them to help. If they are far away, find surrogates. Maybe you can do everything better than Dad or the in-laws. But nothing has to be perfect. *You* don't need to be perfect. You need to be healthy.

You can actively encourage nighttime sleep schedules when your baby is neurologically ready. An infant is usually ready to extend the longest block of sleep into the nighttime hours by around three months. You can encourage this on day 1, however, by being most active in the day and avoiding the temptation to use bright light and playtime during the night.

Try not to let the baby sleep more than three hours at a stretch during the day. Ease the major feeding schedule to the daytime as well. You might want to wake the baby for a feeding and a diaper change right before your bedtime; he or she will be full, dry, and likely to sleep for several hours (and so will you) before the next feeding. And be patient. Infants pick up your cues of anxiety too. Don't let that get in the way of good nighttime habits.

Sleep schedules are important for *us,* too, even if it seems impossible to keep to one. I can't emphasize enough about setting yourself a consistent wake-up time. This anchors your own sleep schedule, even if you nap. Make sure both of you are exposed to enough bright light, so your bodies know when it's day or night (even if you have to be awake in the early hours in a baby's first few months for feedings). Use dim lights (five-watt night-lights, strategically placed) when you need to get up during the night. Make sure night-lights don't shine directly on the crib. If you want to breast-feed but also get more sleep, express your milk so that your partner can do a share of middle-of-the-night feedings. Don't forget the Four Rs of Sleep.

Be sure to look over the tips in Chapter 8 for helping toddlers and teens sleep better. Remember, if you adopt bad habits for *yourself* during the early childbearing years, they may stick with you long after the kids have grown.

Bottom line: Get help, get sleep, and relax and enjoy your baby. Babyhood flies by far too fast.

depression may not be as apparent. A 1999 study found no evidence that these drugs caused birth defects, in utero deaths, or growth impairment. Please talk to your doctor about these options.

Another postdelivery problem to be aware of is postpartum psychosis. In this disorder a woman may seem fine for two to three days after the birth but soon becomes unpredictable and depressed, hyperactive and irritable, often eating and sleeping very little. She may even hear voices or experience hallucinations "commanding" her to hurt (or even kill) the baby. Postpartum psychosis affects only 1 to 2 of every 1,000 new mothers, but it requires immediate hospitalization. Medications such as lithium and the antipsychotic risperidone (Risperdal) started right after delivery can also help women with prior episodes of postpartum psychosis.

Midlife Sleep

Most surveys show that throughout their middle years, healthy, unstressed women gain more sleep than men and continue to have deeper slow-wave sleep than their male partners. (By age thirty to thirty-five most men start to have much less slow-wave sleep than women.) We begin to average out and meet men sleepwise when we're sixty. But more about that later.

The National Sleep Foundation's Women and Sleep Poll revealed that women nearing menopause or those who'd gone through menopause slept ten minutes less each night, and thirty-four minutes less on weekends. Twenty percent of midlife women slept less than six hours per night, compared with 12 percent of younger women. That's about an hour and a half less per week. More important, this may be your break point when you're already shortchanging your sleep.

The survey also found almost 30 percent of menopausal women reported difficulty falling asleep, compared with 18 percent of pre-menopausal women, and their incidence of early-morning awakenings was twice as high. The number of arousals during the night increases with age in both men and women.

Many of the problems we experience with sleep at this stage of life can be linked to hormonal changes. But a number of other factors can affect our sleep. Research by my colleague Dr. Joan Shaver shows that among midlife women, sleep complaints were not related consistently to menopausal symptoms. In many midlife women reporting poor sleep, high life stress and somatic symptoms, including pain, are more evident than high menopausal symptoms. These women also report high emotional distress including depressed mood. In fact, the incidence of depression increases not during menopause but during perimenopause.

In midlife many of us are redefining our marital relationships or long-term partnerships. The incidence of divorce is higher at this time. And women with marital problems are more likely to have poor sleep, independent of depression.

Part of your midlife reassessment may be switching careers or jobs (not always voluntarily). However, many women find themselves working in their later years (often in lower-paying, higher-stress service jobs)

Your Midlife Sleep Rx

With so many special stresses and life situations affecting us at this critical juncture, how can we get a good night's sleep? For one thing, we need to make an extra effort to follow good sleep hygiene. You've heard it before, but it bears repeating:

• Keep a regular wake-up time and try to go to bed no more than an hour earlier or later than your usual turn-in time.

• Avoid caffeine, alcohol, and tobacco at least three hours before bedtime. Try herbal teas instead (see the box on page 103).

• Set up a relaxation period before bed (listen to music, read, have a hot bath). Establish a soothing ritual.

• Maintain a dark, quiet, cool, and safe environment for sleeping.

• Avoid looking at clocks or other time cues during the night.

• If you must get up at night to go to the bathroom, try not to turn on any lights, or at least nothing brighter than a five-watt night-light.

• To reduce stress, learn some relaxation techniques. This may be the perfect time of life to take up yoga or meditation. If you're experiencing any depression, talk to your doctor about therapy, medication, or both. There's no reason to suffer needlessly.

• Get regular exercise; it will help you sleep. Recent studies also show that exercise can help women fight off midlife weight gain, build muscle mass (which burns calories more efficiently), reduce their risk of heart disease, and help keep bones strong. If you've always wanted to learn to ice-skate, play tennis, or golf, it's not too late. But exercise no later than two to three hours before bedtime.

• If you are caring for an ailing or aging relative, investigate day programs and respite care so you can have time for yourself.

Inquire about Meals on Wheels or services provided by religious centers. Try to nap during your downtime.

• Any activity that you find pleasurable will help lessen stress in your life.

• Make an effort to keep up your social connections. Studies show that the more social supports we have, and the more varied they are, the stronger our immune responses will be. Dr. Sheldon Cohen of Carnegie Mellon University in Pittsburgh has found that having diverse social ties—including friends, family, social groups, or religious communities—makes people less susceptible to stress and illness (especially the common cold!), lessens the risk of depression and anxiety, and helps people recuperate faster after illness or injury. All of which can help you sleep better.

• If you're experiencing trouble sleeping, keep a sleep-wake log over a two-week period (see page 163 for a sample). Don't forget to jot down the medications you're taking and any stressful situations or activities you're involved in. Take the diary to your physician and discuss it. If hot flashes are keeping you awake, consider hormone replacement therapy or herbal remedies (see page 74) for a short period.

out of economic necessity. The U.S. Labor Department estimates that by the year 2005 over half of women aged fifty-five to sixty-four will still be in the labor force. Stress and burnout can be lingering problems and these can leach into our sleep lives, disrupting our rest.

Some women who have chosen to stay home and rear children have the freedom at midlife to pursue educational and career goals put on hold years earlier. We may love the intellectual stimulation, but the stress and anxiety of a new workload can hurt our sleep.

It was once believed that the "empty nest" caused depression in midlife women. In actuality, the "nest" may be overcrowded at this stage of life. Many women choose to have children later in life, and young adults often remain at home longer because of economics. Some adult children move back with their parents after a divorce or economic loss. Then there's the dilemma of women in the "sandwich generation," caring for children and aging parents. Where do you find enough time for sleep? The overfull nest can be extremely stressful.

Every time we look in the mirror, we're confronted with the fact that we're getting older. In our youth-oriented society, age is rarely equated with wisdom. Many women view menopause as a time of loss and fading beauty. Studies at the Center for Women's Health Research at the University of Washington, Seattle, have found that negative feelings about aging, when combined with stressful life circumstances and poor health status, worsen stress and depression.

This is also a time in life, unfortunately, when health problems begin to crop up, such as arthritis, osteoarthritis, fibromyalgia, and heart disease. Sleep disorders may emerge in midlife, among them obstructive sleep apnea (often related to postmenopausal weight gain and hormonal changes), restless legs syndrome and periodic leg movement syndrome, and overactive bladder. If you're feeling very sleepy during the day, look at the symptom checklist on page 117. If you're experiencing any of the problems listed (or your partner reports that you are), consult a physician. (I'll discuss sleep disorders in Chapter 4.) Wondering when and if you can retire and planning financially for that time may also add to stress and depression at midlife. Retirement may be an elusive goal for too many of us, and that anxiety can also ruin our sleep.

If we remember the balls and the seesaw, we can easily see how our sleep and wake systems can become unbalanced by special life stresses during this period. This is compounded by poor sleep habits.

Please remember that sleep disruption can be a symptom of depression. Women who've had bouts of major depression during their younger years may be at risk for a recurrence during perimenopause. A 1999 study at the University of Pittsburgh found that women with past depressions had more perceived stress, low mood, and physical symptoms such as headaches, joint pain and stiffness, and vaginal dryness than women who'd never suffered depression. African American women reported more hot flashes and palpitations and fewer depressed moods. (Studies also show that the number one symptom of depression

Sleep Better with Herbal Teas

Herbal teas can be incredibly soothing in the evening and can help you sleep. For one thing, most don't contain any caffeine. That's great for older women who find themselves sensitive to caffeine. Try commercial brands including fruit teas (like raspberry and orange), mint teas, and spiced teas. Other kinds of herbal teas (or herbs that can be made into teas) can be found in natural foods stores. Experiment.

Some herbal teas have properties that specifically aid sleep. For example, a cup or two of valerian tea in the evening may calm anxiety and help you sleep; valerian acts as a "natural" sedative (again, it may take a few weeks to start working). Three to four cups of fragrant chamomile tea a day can also help relieve insomnia.

Other herbal teas may help with hormone-related complaints: Dandelion tea acts as a mild diuretic and may help relieve bloating from PMS (as well as symptoms of bladder infections). Tea brewed from juniper berries is supposed to be good for PMS. Ginger tea may help ease menstrual cramps (it's also said to be helpful for colds and flu). Ginseng tea is said to ease depression, fatigue, and stress, problems that often crop up during the premenstrual period, in perimenopause, and in later life.

You can buy many of these herbal teas packed in tea bags, but purists say it's best to brew from bulk herbs such as flowers, leaves, roots, or barks (aromatics such as chamomile flowers have a shelf life of three to six months; roots can stay fresh up to a year). There are two ways to make herbal tea. You can make an "infusion" by pouring boiling water over the herbs and allowing the tea to steep for five to ten minutes before straining. Or you can make a decoction by simmering an herb bark or root in water for fifteen to thirty minutes, then straining. (For specific types of herbal teas used for various problems, see the chart on pages 78–80.) Don't forget to tell your doctor if you're trying teas from the health food store that aren't commercially packaged.

Fruit and spiced teas can be delicious (add lemon for zing or honey for sweetness); the tastes of other herbs aren't everyone's cup of tea. But you may find the benefits more than make up for a sometimes bitter brew.

among African American women is loss of appetite; they also report dizziness, headaches, and gastrointestinal distress, rather than the classic sadness and loss of self-esteem associated with depression.) So if you're not sleeping well and have puzzling physical problems, don't overlook a recurrence of depression as a possible cause.

A Sounder Sleep in Later Life

It's a myth that we need less sleep the older we get. As we age, our ability to sleep changes, but our need to sleep does *not*. As we get older, there's a natural shift in our biological clock. During most of our adult life, our internal clock triggers sleepiness around 10:00 or 11:00 P.M. (at least for most of us) and wakefulness around 7:00 A.M. But as we age, the clock shifts and we start to feel sleepy several hours earlier, around 7:00 P.M., and the biological clock sounds an unwelcome wake-up call at around 3:00 or 4:00 A.M. It's not clear why this occurs.

It's likely that we get less exposure to light in later life (depriving our inner clock of important cues) because we're less active out-of-doors. Studies suggest that we need at least two hours in natural sunlight to keep our biological clock running smoothly. Unfortunately, studies at Cornell University found that elderly women averaged only forty-five minutes of sunlight per day (those in institutions got a scant two minutes). Other studies suggest that our slowed metabolism and lessened activity in later life could inhibit the natural rise and fall of core body temperature, further messing up our normal sleep signals.

Women do continue to have more slow-wave sleep than men, and women actually sleep more consolidatedly. Additionally, women hold on to their circadian timing longer than men. This may indicate that sleep disturbances in women are influenced more by the homeostatic sleep propensity. Men are noted to spend more time in bed. Could this mean we maintain our sleep health longer and essentially enter "old" age later? I hope so!

Unfortunately, many other health issues tend to disrupt our normal sleep. The most prominent of these is depression. More women than men complain of depression across the years, and depression, as we have seen, affects sleep. Depression tends to increase sleep fragmentation and wakes us up earlier in the morning. A study by the National Institute on Aging found that people who are depressed are three times more likely to report symptoms of insomnia than those who are not depressed.

Depression in later life often coexists with, or is brought on by, chronic illness or disability, such as cancer or heart disease. However, depression needs to be treated as a separate entity. Please see the box on page 106 for a checklist of symptoms of depression. If this sounds like you, see a mental health professional right away. Depression is treatable, and you don't need to go through it without hope or help.

Arthritic pain may be the most common cause of secondary sleep disturbance; people with rheumatoid arthritis report a 60 percent greater prevalence of sleep disorders. The natural movements you make while asleep (as frequently as every ten minutes) may produce joint or muscle pain that wakes you up, and many older people find it harder to get back to sleep. Respiratory problems, such as chronic obstructive pulmonary disease (COPD), can also cause wakefulness.

Heart disease also contributes to sleep problems. In a survey in Sweden examining almost four thousand women with cardiac disease, 18 percent claimed to have poor sleep. Within that group, poor sleep was associated with chest pain and irregular heartbeat. Of course we don't know which comes first, poor sleep or pain. However, in another study, women with coronary artery disease showed a higher incidence of sleep apnea.

Sleep apnea remains a significant predictor of disease even when things like age, smoking status, weight, hypertension (high blood pressure), and diabetes are accounted for. Further, after cardiac surgery women's sleep patterns are greatly disrupted. That disruption improves even in the first postoperative week but can continue over six months. And, finally, patients with hypertension have found their blood pressure rising following sleep deprivation.

Older people are also more likely to be taking several medications, some of which can interfere with sleep or cause interactions that do.

Women who drink or smoke are more likely to have sleep difficulties. One patient of mine, a stylishly dressed eighty-year-old woman whom I'll call Harriet, came to see me complaining of chronic insomnia. Harriet said she was unable to get to sleep quickly. Some nights it took her a very

---

Symptoms of Late-Life Depression

Classic symptoms of late-life depression include

- Withdrawal
- Loss of interest in
  normal activities
- Tearfulness
- Fixation on pain or disease

- Weight loss
- Sleep problems
- Preoccupation with
  death
- Suicidal thoughts

---

long time, and then she found herself sleepy all day long. But as we delved into her history, it became quite obvious that hers was a lifestyle problem, not a problem with changing sleep patterns caused by aging.

Harriet told me that she was sleepy all morning because she didn't fall asleep until very late the night before. She pushed herself to wake up at 9:00 A.M. to listen to a favorite talk show but frequently fell asleep before it was over and might not wake up fully until noon. She did her chores around the house feeling very groggy and often missed out on the volunteer work she loved.

By the afternoon Harriet was feeling quite chipper, and she went out in the evening with her friends. In fact, she was out five nights a week, attending the theater or the ballet, or doing something active with her friends. They ate dinner at approximately 11:00 P.M., or whenever the activity ended. Dinner might include alcohol, and it was topped off with coffee, espresso, or cappuccino. Harriet got home around 1:00 A.M. Then she took a bath and often found it difficult to fall asleep until about 5:00 A.M. The cycle began again, because she really didn't awaken until noon. Now I applaud anyone of eighty who has such an active lifestyle and social circle. But Harriet was sabotaging her own sleep with alcohol, caffeine, and late-night activity, and expecting to fall directly asleep after an exciting evening. Harriet was unusual for her age in a number of ways. She had a severe phase delay schedule—going to bed too late—whereas most elderly people suffer from phase advance problems, going to bed too *early.*

Harriet didn't want to give up her evenings out with her friends, and I wouldn't want her to. So we decided to compromise. We discussed

---

Common Medications That Can Interfere with Sleep

Here are some common drugs more likely to be prescribed for older people which may hamper sleep.

- Antihypertensives (Propanolol)
- Some chemotherapy agents
- Cholesterol-lowering drugs (such as Mevacor)
- Corticosteroids (for rheumatoid arthritis)
- Parkinson's drugs (levodopa)
- Replacement thyroid hormones (high doses)
- Sleeping pills (can cause rebound insomnia when stopped)

---

coming home earlier in the evening, eating dinner at a more normal time (having a pretheater dinner rather than a late-night supper), and consuming little or no alcohol and no caffeine after noon.

Taking a bath in the morning rather than at night allowed her to get to sleep earlier. She needed eight hours of sleep, so if she got to bed at 1:00 A.M., she could get up at 9:00 and be more rested for her day, getting back to the volunteer work she finds so fulfilling. I also suggested that she get out into the daylight (or turn on bright lights) as soon as she woke up to help reset her biological clock. Many older people suffering from dementia find themselves sleeping more in the day rather than at night. If they live alone they may feel unsafe at night. We also see other safety issues arising at this time. Some women can't see or balance well, or they may have some cognitive decline. A woman in the sandwich generation may find her mother wandering the house at night, turning on the stove or calling out for her because she cannot sleep. (This is usually a sign of dementia.) Sometimes the problem gets so bad that concerned caregivers opt for assisted living or a nursing home facility for their loved ones. But this change may make things worse.

Most institutions encourage residents to turn in early. "Better" facilities provide areas where nighttime gatherings and food are available, reinforcing a schedule of nighttime activity and abnormal sleep patterns. Conversely, too many places allow daytime napping and inactivity, which can worsen things even further.

Many elderly people lose their external cues for normal circadian rhythms and revert to an infant's sleep pattern. We can change that and reinforce good rhythms if we wish, but it requires a lot of dedication on the part of the institution or caregiver. Light is the most important signal to our biological clock and, as I mentioned, older people often live in an environment that isn't bright enough; institutions are notoriously poorly lit.

Dr. Sonia Ancoli-Israel, a professor of psychiatry at the University of California, San Diego, and author of *All I Want Is a Good Night's Sleep* (Mosby, 1996), has carried out significant research to show that bright light therapy and activity can improve the sleep-wake patterns of nursing home residents. She assigned students to patients to keep them active and alert all day as well. Light helped—but activities which did not reinforce alertness did not. This personal attention isn't always possible. However, before getting too worried about yourself or a loved one, see if light and activity can make an early difference.

Women (*and* men) who live in assisted living facilities or nursing homes may experience sundowning. This phenomenon involves an evening (sundown) onset of confusion and frequently irritability, agitation, or delirium. You can tell the difference between a simple lessening of circadian rhythm and sundowning by the severity of symptoms. A sundowner gets much worse in the evening, experiencing general confusion and lack of attention (although some new research indicates this agitated behavior also occurs during the day, but is more often noticed at night). The treatment for this problem similarly requires more daytime activities and bright lights. However, in severe cases, a doctor might prescribe an antipsychotic medication at night.

I must emphasize that both of these conditions are more behavioral than organic. However, with Alzheimer's disease or some other organic form of senility, there are real changes in brain function that can affect the ability to sleep. Fragmented sleep occurs early in the course of Alzheimer's. In fact, for some patients we see little difference in the brain waves on an electroencephalogram (EEG) among the three states of consciousness, wake, NREM, or REM sleep. That's why the circadian markers of schedule and light are so important. They give what is left of the sleep system a boost. Medications may also be needed.

Sleep Tips for Midlife and Beyond

- Get out in the sunlight once a day for at least one to two hours.
- Don't keep home lighting too dim.
- Set a regular wake time, and keep it constant (napping can disrupt your biological clock later in life).
- Exercise regularly. The best times are late afternoon and early evening.
- Try yoga or other relaxation techniques.
- Avoid caffeine after noon.
- Accept help. It's not a sign of weakness.
- Get a good physical; ask about hormones and supplements.
- Check out medications as possible sleep disrupters.
- Be your own sleep investigator. Keep a sleep log (see the sample on page 163) to match episodes of bad sleep with habits and stressful events.
- If you find yourself experiencing a depressed mood (or any symptoms of depression), don't hesitate to seek a therapist. Remember, illness, disability, and depression often go hand in hand.
- Plan a happy future, be optimistic, and seek changes where they're needed (career, relationships, activities, lifestyle).

Overactive Bladder

Why is it that, as we get older, we seem to have to "go" more in the middle of the night?

I'm sure you wonder why you can go all day and hardly have to visit the bathroom, but the second you get into bed, you have the urge to go. As we age, the vascular system and kidneys may function less efficiently. So during the day, when we're standing up or walking around, fluids may accumulate in the legs or ankles, causing swelling. But when we lie down in bed, the fluids go back into circulation and are sent to the kidneys. Presto! A wake-up call in the middle of the night.

As I mentioned in Chapter 1, sometimes nighttime trips to the bathroom aren't the result of a full bladder and an urge to pee but are simply prompted by a thought that arises because we've woken up: "I'm awake, I might as well go to the bathroom." This can become a habit. A similar cycle occurs in people with significant sleep apnea (see page 132). So, again, the first thing you have to do is change that habit. Keep telling yourself that you don't really have to urinate, and that you can go back to sleep. I assure you, this does seem to work for many people.

But there are exceptions. Millions of them, actually. Some 17 million Americans (most of them women) suffer from an overactive bladder, uncontrollable urges to urinate so sudden that they often don't make it to the bathroom on time. When that happens urine leaks out and you have urge incontinence.

What's going on is a short circuit in the messages the bladder sends to the brain. Normally, as the bladder fills and expands, nerve endings signal the brain that the bladder is full. But the sphincter muscles surrounding the bladder neck and urethra stay shut until we get to a bathroom and "tell" the bladder to empty. When we know it's okay to go, the bladder wall contracts and the sphincter muscles relax, allowing urine to flow. But in women with overactive bladder, this message gets sent long before the bladder is full, and the sphincter relaxes before we're ready.

The short circuit can be caused or aggravated by nerve problems (in the brain, spinal cord, or bladder itself), by weakness in the pelvic floor muscles that support the bladder or muscles in the urethra, and by caffeine, alcohol, or acidic or spicy foods, which irritate the bladder. Medications can also irritate the bladder. Not surprisingly, drinking too much fluid at night can make the problem worse, although drinking does not necessarily cause it.

Sometimes eliminating caffeine and alcohol along with spicy and acidic foods (such as citrus fruits, tomato juice, and vinegar) can help. Consciously retraining your bladder to hold urine for longer periods may be recommended, along with controlling fluid intake (especially in the evening). Two medications, tolterodine (Detrol) and oxybutynin (Ditropan), work on brain chemicals to help control the abnormal signals from the bladder. However, Ditropan can also cause dry mouth, a problem for some older women; Detrol has less strong effects on salivary glands. Ask your doctor if these medications can help you.

A last resort is surgery to implant a bladder "pacemaker," a tiny electrical device called InterStim, which sends impulses to the bladder to prompt it to function more normally. In clinical trials InterStim reduced trips to the bathroom as well as incontinence. There are different remedies for incontinence, including collagen implants to help the urethra form a stronger seal and surgery to correct problems caused by weakened pelvic floor muscles, but these will not help overactive bladder or restore sleep.

However, some experts do recommend Kegel exercises to strengthen the muscles that support the bladder neck and urethra. Pelvic floor muscles are often weakened by childbirth and lack of estrogen after menopause. Kegels can not only help with mild stress incontinence (where you leak urine when there's pressure on the bladder, such as during exercise or coughing or sneezing) but also initiate a reflex that relaxes the bladder and decreases the urge to urinate.

Here's the basic technique for doing Kegel exercises:

• Locate the muscles you need to contract. While you're urinating, consciously pull up and in on muscles to stop the flow of urine. These are the muscles that support the bladder neck and urethra.

• For the exercise itself, contract the pelvic floor muscles as hard as you can (without tightening the buttocks or bearing down) and hold that contraction for at least ten seconds.

• As you contract your muscles, exhale gently through your mouth to keep from straining. Rest between contractions.

• Start with ten repetitions at least ten times a day, then gradually increase the number and frequency over six weeks. You need to keep doing Kegels to maintain pelvic floor strength and prevent (or minimize) urine leakage.

Some older women may have nerve damage in the pelvic floor area, and their muscles may not respond to efforts to contract them. Electrical stimulation, with an intravaginal device or a special chair, can help.

Any way you stop or reduce those nighttime wake-up calls can clearly help you get a better night's sleep!

Your Later-Life Sleep Rx
(or Retiring After Retirement)

Many older people unknowingly throw off their biological clock when they retire. Since most don't have to be at an office, they sleep later. They may nap during the day. They may keep their homes too dimly lit (sometimes to save money, sometimes because of sensitivity to bright light). They may go to bed earlier than they did before—and wonder why they're waking up so early! While I've recommended napping for younger women, in later life naps can disrupt the biological clock and sleep-wake patterns. So my recommendation is *not* to nap.

Exposure to bright light can help reset your biological clock. For older people this may mean following the sun rather than working with a light box. For one thing, light therapy may be very difficult for those with eye diseases or sensitivity to bright light. The sun at dawn is actually equal to a bright light box and probably more acceptable, if your environment is safe. So an early-morning walk can not only foster a better sleep-wake schedule but also provide valuable exercise. And it helps you get outdoors, where you can meet other people and stay engaged in the world, rather than being isolated and inactive.

Hot baths can also help sleep. You'll recall that taking a hot bath (in water that's at least 100 degrees Fahrenheit) a couple of hours before bedtime for at least thirty minutes aids sleep by first raising body temperature, then lowering it once you lie down in a cool room. This helps you fall asleep faster and sleep more deeply. In fact, studies show that hot baths are as good as (or better than) benzodiazepines for aiding sleep in older people. (Again, if you have high blood pressure or a heart condition, or are prone to dizziness, don't take very hot baths without talking with your doctor.)

Don't forget sleep-inducing bedtime snacks, especially milk. (Milk, bananas, cheese, and even turkey all contain tryptophan, a chemical that helps sleep, see page 39). If you suffer from gastrointestinal reflux, using six- to eight-inch blocks to elevate the head of your bed can prevent stomach acid from leaking out. You may also consider medications that inhibit production of stomach acid at bedtime.

Many older patients ask me about melatonin. Remember, healthy seniors do not have less melatonin, so attempting to replace it with supplements is not a good idea. For one thing, melatonin production is controlled internally. Second, most available dose levels of commercially prepared melatonin are much higher than the body normally produces. Melatonin also acts to constrict smooth muscle tissue (such as in artery walls). In people with arteries already narrowed by cholesterol-laden plaques, it can exacerbate high blood pressure and impair blood flow to the heart, causing angina. So don't take melatonin if you have cardiovascular disease. In any case, melatonin's effects are modest at best, affecting only the onset of sleep, not how long you sleep. There are *no* long-term studies of effectiveness and safety of melatonin in humans.

Use sleep medications very cautiously, if at all. For one thing, your metabolism slows as you age, so you may not metabolize the standard dose as fast and the effects can last longer, causing side effects not unlike a morning hangover, along with confusion and balance problems. Studies also show that the use of sleeping pills can increase the risk of falls among older people. Frequently, older people may forget they've already taken a dose of sleeping medication and take another pill.

For women experiencing sundowning, combining exercise with light in the late afternoon can help. This discipline is especially good for the elderly, whose circadian rhythms seem to be shortened. Walking outside before sunset helps you get not only stimulating exercise but a good dose of bright light, and will help retard sleep onset from a too-early 8:00 or 9:00 P.M. to 11:00 P.M., which will result in a more normal wake time.

Exercise has many benefits in later life, including helping you obtain a better night's sleep. Women who engage in moderate activities, like walking, gardening, or bowling, four or more times a week, live longer than sedentary women. Women who exercise only once a week live longer than those who do not. Strength training with light weights (which builds muscle mass) can improve endurance and help prevent falls.

Depression is not a "normal" part of aging, and it's very treatable at any age. But according to the American Association of Geriatric Psychiatry, fewer than half of older people experiencing depression are being diagnosed correctly, and half of those who *are* properly diagnosed aren't getting treatment. If you find yourself experiencing vague physical complaints, low moods, and insomnia, see your doctor.

Women with Parkinson's disease often find sleep more difficult. Although the tremors associated with Parkinsonism disappear in sleep, muscle tone is elevated in REM sleep. Remember, in REM sleep we are in a state of muscle atonia (paralyzed) and cannot act out our dreams. Well, increased muscle tone in REM sleep allows us to move and attempt to carry out the dream activity. So, women with Parkinson's disease may have REM behavior disorder. Treatments include doses of levodopa or Benadryl, which is also mildly sedating. For some people the benzodiazepine Klonopin (clonazepam, in doses of 0.5 milligram per hour of sleep) at bedtime is helpful to prevent these movements and ensure sleep. Sleep itself also helps people with Parkinson's disease, so avoid sleep deprivation.

Again, stay active. Volunteering is a great way to get out and meet new people, keep mentally fit, and reduce stress. Studies at Duke University and elsewhere show that among older people regular attendance at church, synagogue, or mosque can improve health (and even reduce the chances of dying after a heart attack!).

Speaking of keeping your mind active, many local colleges and universities offer courses for older people. Contrary to popular belief, we don't lose our mental abilities as we age. We may have the occasional slip in memory ("Where *did* I put those keys?"), but many skills actually get sharper. Recent studies show the brain grows new cells throughout life. So don't let those new neurons go to waste! Train them and get them organized for better sleep!

4

Women and Sleep Disorders
When Sleep Won't Come

Occasional problems with sleep can be upsetting, but most of the time they resolve themselves. However, if you're having trouble with sleep on a regular basis, or you are excessively sleepy in the daytime most days of the week, it may be a sign that you've got a sleep disorder.

Approximately seventy-five types of sleep disorders have been identified, ranging from sleep apnea to narcolepsy. However, according to the National Sleep Foundation, only 4 percent of adults who experience frequent sleep problems see a doctor for advice or treatment. So every night millions of people are suffering needlessly.

While effective treatments for sleep disorders are available at specialized sleep centers, many of us don't know the symptoms or don't have a health care provider who does. Amazingly, nearly two-thirds of adults have never known their physician to ask this simple question: "How have you been sleeping lately?"

One of the reasons is that sleep medicine is not taught in medical schools (and what sleep textbooks there are don't even discuss the special concerns of women). Although my colleagues and I have all done a lot of local teaching, particularly about sleep apnea and narcolepsy, your physician may not be aware of your specific disorder. So you need to find out all you can. There are many books, Web sites, and other sources of information out there (and you'll find the best ones in Appendix II). I encourage you to share this information with your health care provider and seek specialized care when it's needed (see Appendix III).

Is It a Sleep Disorder?

Symptoms of Insomnia

- Difficulty falling asleep
- Difficulty staying asleep
- Early-morning awakening
- Waking up feeling unrefreshed

Symptoms of Obstructive Sleep Apnea

- Loud snoring, snorting, gasping
- Restless, nonrestorative sleep
- Excessive daytime sleepiness

Symptoms of Restless Legs Syndrome

- An urge to move limbs
- Uncomfortable "crawling" sensations in legs or arms
- Motor restlessness
- Worsening of these symptoms when you're trying to relax

Symptoms of Periodic Limb Movement Syndrome

- Repetitive, stereotyped movements of limbs during sleep that occur every fifteen to forty seconds
- Movements usually involving the toe, with flexing at the ankle, knee, or hip
- Increased symptoms with alcohol use, pregnancy, age
- Daytime sleepiness

Symptoms of Narcolepsy

- Profound, sudden, and unavoidable daytime sleepiness
- Sudden loss of muscle tone during laughter, anger, or excitement (cataplexy)
- Hallucinations while fighting off a strong urge to sleep
- Fragmented nighttime sleep
- Sleep paralysis

Do You Suspect You Have a Sleep Disorder?

If you have several of the symptoms listed on page 117, the first thing to do is begin to keep track of when you get sleepy during the day. Is it in the afternoon? If so, try to add fifteen to thirty minutes to your planned sleep time each night. Things should be better (if not perfect) after six nights. Add more time as needed. If that doesn't work, something may be disrupting your sleep.

Do you get sleepy soon after waking and stay that way all day? Ask your partner about your nighttime habits. Are you snoring? Are you kicking the sheets off? If so, see your physician. You may have a sleep disorder, so no matter how much you sleep you simply do not wake up refreshed.

If you suffer from insomnia, start keeping a sleep log (see page 163) to see if you uncover any bad habits that may be causing the problem.

Are you doing everything right to structure your sleep and find yourself still sleepy? See your physician for a checkup. Your sleepiness could be the result of a change in thyroid function, anemia, or other undiagnosed health problems.

A sleep disorder means you consistently have difficulty with sleep— either too much or too little—or strange things happen when you sleep. Typically, your symptoms are frequent; you wouldn't have symptoms two days a month, they would occur almost every day. If your symptoms come and go, you might very well think first about your normal hormonal cycle or poor sleep habits.

Insomnia: The Common Cold of Sleep Problems

By far the most common sleep problem among women is insomnia. The National Sleep Foundation Women and Sleep Poll found that over half of women report symptoms of insomnia (difficulty falling or staying asleep) during any given month.

Insomnia is usually a *symptom* of another, underlying problem. For women, as I've mentioned, this can be hidden depression or anxiety, pain syndromes like fibromyalgia or headaches, the effects of pregnancy, symptoms of premenstrual syndrome and perimenopause, menopausal

---

Health Problems That Can Affect Sleep

- Depression
- Anxiety
- Under- or overactive thyroid
- Anemia
- Arthritis pain
- Fibromyalgia
- Coronary artery disease
- Angina
- Irregular heartbeat
- Hypertension
- Chronic obstructive pulmonary disease
- Obstructive sleep apnea
- Asthma
- Alzheimer's disease
- Parkinson's disease

---

hot flashes, or an overactive bladder. In some cases insomnia can be caused by behaviors (like irregular sleep habits or too much caffeine) or environmental factors, like noise. Insomnia can also be a symptom of other sleep disorders, such as restless legs. And it can be caused by medical problems, including breathing difficulties resulting from asthma and chronic obstructive pulmonary disorder, an overactive thyroid, Parkinson's disease, or other movement disorders. Women with chronic fatigue syndrome often have trouble getting to sleep. In fact, their overwhelming fatigue is not relieved by sleep. Most psychiatric disorders are associated with some alteration in sleep.

Women with insomnia frequently complain of the inability to function well and reduced quality of life. Despite feeling fatigued all day, few can nap. Too often a cycle of worry over sleep keeps you awake at night. You have a sleepless night and say to yourself, "Boy, I hope I sleep better tonight." You might even go to bed extra early to "capture" more sleep. But disrupting your normal sleep pattern can lead to early awakening . . . and more worry over sleeplessness.

This is a perfect time to recall those balls on the seesaw. By worrying about sleep during our waking hours, we enlarge that wake ball with anxiety, try to sleep at a time when our sleep system is not ready (thereby reducing the effect of the sleep ball), and wonder why we can't cure a simple problem. Day by day, the balls get further out of balance and we suffer more symptoms of insomnia. That's why my first questions to an insomniac are, When did it start? What was happening in your life? and What remedies did you choose? The answers to those questions can suggest a simple course of treatment, or they may uncover underlying problems.

Take one of my patients, whom I'll call Molly, now in her fifties. She was a daytime napper for years. She told me, "It started when my son was born and needed night feedings. My sleep got interrupted, and I began a habit of napping in the day. I always kept an ear out for my children at night, in case they should need me, so I never slept very well. When my kids started dating, I waited up for them to get in. Now they're in college, and I still can't sleep through the night. So I just keep taking naps."

Sounds like a simple situation, right? Tell Molly to cut out the naps and do all her sleeping at night. But it's not quite as simple as that. First, Molly had to decide if it mattered whether she slept through the night. After all, she'd managed all these years with daytime napping. Second, Molly had to decide if she wanted to go through the discomfort of compressed and insufficient sleep while we tried to reorganize her sleep schedule. Ultimately, Molly chose to try it, because she wanted to make use of her newfound freedom to resume the career she'd interrupted to have children.

Sleep Restriction Therapy

In order to reorganize Molly's sleep, we used a technique called sleep restriction therapy, developed by Dr. Arthur Speilman at the City University of New York. It can be very effective for insomnia.

First, we looked at how much total sleep Molly had been getting over a twenty-four-hour period and compressed her time in bed to that many hours. She chose a consistent wake-up time, and we backed up her bedtime to encompass that many hours of sleep. We forbade daytime napping. When Molly was consistently sleeping the designated number of hours for at least a week, she was allowed to increase her sleep time by fifteen minutes. Then she held to that amount of time for a set period, adding fifteen-minute increments until she was consistently sleeping most of the night.

As an example, Molly slept about five hours at night and one or two hours during some days. Therefore, we selected a nighttime sleep period of six hours to start. Molly chose 7:00 A.M. as her wake time. So she was not allowed to go to bed until 1:00 A.M.! (7 minus 6 equals 1). Once she slept consistently from 1:00 to 7:00 A.M. for a week, she was able to go to bed fifteen minutes earlier, to sleep from 12:45 until 7:00 A.M. Again, she held to this time until she slept consistently for a week, then rolled back to 12:30. Since she also had to give up her naps, she was tired in the beginning. I just asked her to be careful and to try to avoid activities that require full attention, like driving. After about a month Molly was able to sleep well between midnight and 7:00 A.M. She was quite pleased.

Actually, Molly's problem, caused by sleep habits acquired when her children were young, is not uncommon. Some women accept disturbed sleep (and the steps they take to deal with it) as part of parenthood. Once the kids are grown, however, women may be more bothered by their disturbed sleep and seek medical attention (especially if, like Molly, they want to return to work).

As problems are more complex, solutions get more complicated, too.

Another of my patients, Janine, who's in her thirties, told me that her insomnia started during her college years, when she'd lie awake nights thinking and planning her life. That kind of nighttime ruminating became a habit. Janine came to me after she'd been married for six years. Both she and her husband had high-powered careers. Both were chronically overworked, trying to save enough money to buy a house and start a family. At the same time they were faced with helping his parents, who were ailing. Any free time they might have had over the weekends was taken up with her in-laws, and Janine seldom had private time with her spouse to enjoy activities they used to share, like biking. Their sex life became almost nonexistent. And she worried about it all. Janine came to the sleep center in tears, complaining that her insomnia was worse than it had ever been.

In this case we could tie sleeplessness to stress and depression. Not to blame the victim, but Janine had worried herself into inactivity, depression, and sleeplessness. We planned a simple attack on worrying (she started a worry book, described on page 27), and we discussed ways to improve her sleep habits. I also helped Janine realize that depression was a large part of her problem. She needed counseling and antidepressant medications to help with the other aspects of her treatment.

If we think about the sleep seesaw, it's easy to see how depression can unbalance the balls. Our brains use the same chemicals and neurotransmitters for sleep as they do for mood. An imbalance in chemicals can affect both. In Janine's case, restoring the chemical balance with antidepressants relieved the symptoms of depression, which was a major underlying cause of her insomnia. However, we also needed to take steps to rebalance her sleep and wake systems and restore balance to her waking hours, making free time for pleasurable activities and exercise. If your life is out of balance, your sleep will be, too.

Sleep Potions:
The Good, the Bad, and the Ugly

Let's start by remembering those balls on the seesaw. Any remedy that reduces daytime alertness and stress will help the sleep system get in balance. Similarly, anything that strengthens the sleep system will allow it to counter that old wake system.

Let's go over the difference between the good, the bad, and the ugly sleep potions in general terms. Good sleep potions are those that work for you! If they're medications, they're ones your doctor prescribed for you. Bad potions are things you choose *without* consulting a health specialist, such as over-the-counter drugs and herbs. The ugly potions are things that are damaging, like alcohol, pot, and drugs prescribed for someone else (perhaps a friend offers to give you a few of her sleeping tablets). A big, bad no-no.

Think about it: Your doctor knows about your general health and

W O M E N   A N D   S L E E P   D I S O R D E R S

Antianxiety Drugs Used for Sleep Problems

Brand Name	Generic Name	Dose Range (mg)
Xanax	alprazolam	0.25–0.5 mg 3 times a day
Valium	diazepam	2–10 mg
Ativan	lorazepam	1–4 mg at time of sleep
BuSpar	buspirone	5–10 mg at time of sleep

can keep track of other medications you are taking and their potential side effects. The medications he or she prescribes will be more targeted in your brain and doing the job you need.

When you grab an over-the-counter medication, you're usually using the side effect (sleepiness) of a drug meant for another reason, in this case antihistamines (usually diphenhydramine, which causes drowsiness in many people). Why on earth do we want to use a drug meant for allergies when we're having trouble sleeping? The other issue is that those side effects may compound other illnesses you have and worsen things instead of improve them. Plus, antihistamines can cause dry mouth. So, as far as I'm concerned, with a few exceptions (see page 126), I recommend you skip the Sominex, Nytol, Sleep-Eze, and so on, unless, for some reason, you can't take other sleeping pills. Speak with your health care provider first.

More important: You should *not* try your friend's prescription. What works for one may harm the other. However, a good sleeping potion is food that contains tryptophan, a serotonin-building protein, such as milk or bananas (see page 39).

Here's information on possibly helpful potions.

Antianxiety drugs are very useful for people whose insomnia is caused by racing thoughts and excessive worry. Nonsedating benzodiazepines and the drug BuSpar taken during the day, or antianxiety drugs that promote drowsiness taken at bedtime, can relieve anxiety and help you sleep better at night. Depending on the preparation, some may leave you with a hangover effect in the morning, but generally they are not habit-forming when used correctly.

Sleeping Pills

Brand Name	Generic Name	Class	Duration of Action (hr)	Dose (mg)
Sonata	zaleplon	pyrazolopyridine	1–3 hrs	5–10
Ambien	zolpidem	imidazopyridine	4–5 hrs	5–10
Halcion	triazolam	benzodiazepine	3–4 hrs	0.125–25
ProSom	estazolam	benzodiazepine	6–8 hrs	1
Restoril	temazepam	benzodiazepine	6–8 hrs	15–30
Doral	quazepam	benzodiazepine	8–10 hrs	7.5–15
Dalmane	flurazepam	benzodiazepine	12+ hrs	15–30
Klonopin	clonazepam	benzodiazepine	8–12+ hrs	0.5–2

Sleeping pills used properly can be a great help. But my advice is to take them for the least amount of time necessary and work to improve sleep in other ways. It is important to understand your symptoms of insomnia.

Do you have trouble *falling* asleep? Then take a short-acting sedating drug like triazolam (Halcion), zolpidem (Ambien), or the newest and shortest-acting, zaleplon (Sonata). These drugs remain effective for up to four hours. Subjects using Sonata performed normally even if awakened one hour after administration.

You may remember the controversy over Halcion a few years ago. People were claiming that they had amnesia as a result of the drug (and were doing dangerous things in the night). Well, that's actually possible with *any* drug that sedates you if you awaken during its effective time. You are in a stupor and have little or no memory of your actions, and your balance may be off. Be careful. If you must awaken for child care or bathroom visits, consider Sonata. Otherwise there are few side effects to these drugs.

If, however, your problem is *staying* asleep, you may need a longer-acting drug, such as temazepam (Restoril) or flurazepam (Dalmane). These are sedating benzodiazepines. The problem is that these drugs may still be working when you need to get up in the morning. Sonata has an especially short-acting time (one to three hours). So you could con-

Antidepressants Used for Sleep

Brand Name	Generic Name	Class	Dose (mg)
Desyrel	trazodone	atypical	50–300
Remeron	mirtazapine	piperazinoazepine	15–30
Serzone	nefazodone	mixed uptake inhibitor	100
Sinequan	doxepin	tricyclic	10–70
Elavil	amitriptyline	tricyclic	10–25

ceivably use it again at 3:00 or 4:00 A.M., capture four more hours of sleep, and awaken without that hangover effect.

It is possible to develop a tolerance to these drugs, and find yourself needing increased doses. However, the likelihood is very slim when using the shorter-acting ones. If this happens, consult your physician for an alternate strategy.

Antidepressants: Sometimes physicians will use other classes of drugs, such as antidepressants in low doses, to affect sleep. In such doses, side effects are usually minimal, although they can include dry mouth, light-headedness, and difficulty urinating. If you are suffering from depression, adequate treatment of the depression will help your sleep symptoms. Some of the sedating antidepressants commonly used today include mirtazapine (Remeron), trazodone (Desyrel), and nefazodone (Serzone). As I've stressed throughout this book, it's most important to recognize depression as a source of sleep difficulty and treat the depression thoroughly. The chart above lists popular sedating antidepressant medications, but the doses indicated are for the symptom of insomnia. If you are depressed, chances are your dose will be higher.

Antihistamines: What about things like Tylenol PM? Well, if you're in pain, treating the pain will likely improve your sleep. Tylenol PM is a combination of pain reliever and diphenhydramine, or Benadryl. It is important to understand that all of these over-the-counter sleep potions contain the antihistamine diphenhydramine: Compoz, Hydril, Noradryl, Nytol, Sleep-Eze, Sominex, and Tusstat. Again, these remedies are marginally effective at best and can cause dry mouth, so you may be better served with a short course of prescription medication. So discuss this with your doctor before buying anything at the drugstore.

When You Need a Sleep Aid

As you can imagine, selecting the right medication is a highly individual act. You should choose a doctor who is willing to work with you on the best approach and understand that you may need to try several medications before you're comfortable.

In some instances, medications that aid sleep can be appropriate for short periods. For instance, during a high-stress period like a family illness or divorce, when you just cannot get stress under control, sleeping medications help to take the edge off and provide strength to your sleep system.

Sometimes I recommend that my patients take sleeping medications on a temporary basis while I'm teaching them better sleep habits and sleep restriction. For example, I might suggest that a patient take a short-acting drug like Halcion or Ambien up to three nights a week to give herself control over sleep. I leave it up to my patients to decide which three nights it is absolutely necessary to sleep and take the pills then.

Our sleep center was involved in the early research on Sonata, and the results look especially good for people whose main problem is that they wake in the middle of the night and can't get back to sleep. Taking Sonata would allow them to get those three or four more hours of sleep, then awaken feeling refreshed. It may also allow them to sleep on an "emergency basis" when they would otherwise not be able to, like during the day of jet travel over time zones, or during intermittent shift work.

Again, remember that while using *any* sleeping pill, you may have episodes of amnesia or poor coordination if you awaken and try to function. So choose the nights wisely, and don't take sleep medications on a night during which you may be awakened or are alone with young children.

Your Sleep Rx for Insomnia
(Be Your Own Sleep Doctor)

In many cases, you can be your own sleep doctor if you recognize the behaviors causing your insomnia.

Are you drinking too much caffeine or alcohol? Do you eat dinner too late in the evening? Are you using your bedroom as a home office with piles of files always in plain sight? Do you allow yourself to toss and turn for long periods while you're hoping to drop off? Are you glancing at the bedroom clock every five minutes and worrying about when you'll fall asleep? Do you sleep very late on Saturdays and Sundays, only to find yourself wide awake those nights . . . and sleepy all day Monday?

If you've answered yes to any of these questions, you're setting yourself up for insomnia. Changing your behavior is often the first line of treatment. Recall Dr. Shaver's Four Rs of Sleep:

• **Regularize your sleep-wake patterns.** Set your alarm and get up at the same time every day. Avoid naps, unless they are a regular part of your routine and don't disrupt nighttime sleep. Try to sleep the same number of hours each night. Figure out how much sleep you need to be at your best and stick with it.

• **Ritualize cues for good sleep.** Keep your sleeping environment quiet, dark, cool, and safe for sleeping. Go to bed only when you're sleepy. Use your bedroom only for sleeping and sex. Use soothing routines like hot baths or massage.

• **Relax to control tension.** Assume a comfortable position, clear your mind by stopping disturbing thoughts, and concentrate instead on a relaxing scene, or deep breathing. Practice these techniques so you can help your body relax and prepare for sleep.

• **Resist behaviors that interfere with sleep.** Avoid alcohol, tobacco, and caffeine, as well as heavy meals too close to bedtime.

Make sure you get regular daily exercise. But try not to do it within two or three hours of bed. Get the clock out of sight.

If you think that making such behavioral changes won't help your insomnia as much as taking medication, think again. A 1999 study from Laval University in Quebec compared drug therapy and behavioral therapy in seventy-eight older men and women suffering from insomnia. They were randomized to receive either sleeping pills or an eight-week course in changing sleep behaviors, both therapies, or a placebo. While medications and behavioral therapy were equally effective in the short term, after two years behavioral treatment produced the most improvement in sleep. In fact, a majority of patients who had behavioral therapy no longer even qualified as insomniacs. In contrast, half of those who took medications (either alone or with sleep training) still had insomnia.

For sleep problems tied to hormonal influences, take appropriate action. For premenstrual syndrome, cut down on salt to reduce bloating, restrict caffeine, and take extra calcium. If hot flashes or other menopausal symptoms are keeping you awake, consider estrogen replacement (or new herbal phytoestrogen or soy menopausal supplements). There are many estrogens to choose from these days, including new plant-based conjugated estrogens. You need to take them for only a few years to ease menopausal symptoms. And do try that soy smoothie.

If you find yourself awakening from a sound sleep because of frequent, intense urges to go to the bathroom and then can't fall back to sleep, ask your physician about the new medications for overactive bladder, Detrol and Ditropan. While these medications can cause dry mouth and other side effects, they may help you sleep through the night.

Don't keep tossing and turning. Again, if you can't fall asleep in bed after a reasonable period (say thirty minutes), and are getting upset, get up, go into a darkened or dimly lit room, and do some quiet activity. Read, knit, listen to soothing music (my editor swears by MTV's *After Hours* or VH-1's *Insomniac Music Theater*, although I personally don't find that music soothing). But *don't* use this time to catch up on active or overstimulating tasks like doing the laundry or office paperwork. When you feel drowsy, go back to bed.

If you're having trouble falling asleep, try warming up your feet. Recent studies suggest that inadequate vasodilation (opening of blood vessels to increase blood flow) may be causing some sleep problems. Why? It seems that when we lie down, the body lowers its core temperature and redistributes heat to the periphery. Swiss researchers found this vasodilation one of the best predictors of sleep onset. So tucking a hot water bottle by your feet or slipping on a pair of socks might help you get to sleep more quickly. This remedy might be especially helpful to older women with poor circulation in their feet. It's certainly worth a try!

However, your body shouldn't be overheated. Some people pile on the blankets whether it's summer or winter. We sleep better in a slightly cool environment, so removing that heavy quilt or duvet might help.

Assess your bedding: Is it comfortable? Pillows that are too hard, too soft, or too flat can also interfere with sleep. Even the most expensive pillows go flat eventually. So you may need to spring for some new ones. Are your sheets comfy? Sheets can chafe if they are too rough on your skin; try some unscented fabric softener. Cotton sheets are best; polyester can make you perspire. Mattress manufacturers advise turning the mattress every so often to prevent a permanent groove from forming.

Allergies can interfere with sleep and contribute to stuffy noses and headaches in the morning. So take steps to minimize allergens in the bedroom (see the box on page 131). Here's where antihistamines can be helpful at night. For most people, the worst allergen in the bedroom is dust mites (microscopic organisms that feed off flakes of dead skin). Dust mites regard your mattress and box spring as deluxe accommodations, so use zippered, allergen-proof covers on your pillow, mattress, box spring, and blankets to keep them contained. The most comfortable are non-vinyl coverings that allow water vapor to escape and won't make you perspire. Cover the zipper with fabric-reinforced tape.

Sleep-Related Breathing Problems

Think you don't snore? Ask your partner. The answer may surprise you. Perhaps 40 million Americans are habitual snorers.

Snoring results from relaxation of the throat muscles during sleep and the collapse of excess tissue in the back of the mouth and throat, which partially blocks the upper airway. When this happens, you're forced to inhale more deeply, pulling even more floppy tissue into the airway, causing those tissues (usually the soft palate, pharynx, and uvula) to vibrate. That's the noise you hear.

Snoring is almost always a sign of a compromised airway, which can lead to a spectrum of sleep-disordered breathing. Picture an ice cream cone as the airway. At the top the airway is fully opened; at the bottom it is sealed shut. Air flows through the top easily but not at all through the bottom. In between are changes that make it more and more difficult for air to flow through, and resistance to airflow is increased. When this occurs, the lungs need to suck harder to pull air in. If the suction is strong and the tissues of the airway are floppy, they can be sucked shut. Even if these changes are subtle, they can cause you to arouse or wake briefly from sleep. Depending on how severe the changes are, they may also be associated with decreased oxygen. Together the awakenings and decreases in oxygen affect the quality of your life during waking hours, making you feel sleepy and groggy during the day. The problem of subtle changes in the airway is called upper airway resistance syndrome (UARS). The more severe changes are called obstructive sleep apnea (OSA), a complete closure of the airway so no air can pass (I'll discuss this shortly).

Allergies in the Bedroom

If indoor allergies are interfering with your sleep, the Asthma and Allergy Foundation of America offers the following tips:

- Wash all bedding—pillowcases, sheets, blankets, mattress pad, and comforters (and kids' stuffed animals) in hot water (130°F) every week to kill the dust mites. Warm water washing and hot air drying aren't enough. If you can't wash your comforter once a week, consider an allergen-proof cover.
- Carpeting harbors dust, dust mites, and animal dander (another potent allergen). If possible, replace wall-to-wall carpeting with hardwood floors that can be mopped, and use washable area rugs.
- If possible, replace heavy lined drapes with shades or lightweight washable curtains. Always wash in hot (130°) water.
- Reduce humidity in the bedroom to less than 50 percent using a dehumidifier or an air conditioner. Remember to clean (or replace) filters, and follow manufacturers' cleaning directions to keep them mold-free. (There are special sprays for filters that help trap more dust and other allergens.)
- Air filters can be helpful, but won't remove all allergens from the air. High Efficiency Particulate Air (HEPA) filters trap the smallest particles. Change the filters often. Make sure the unit is quiet and won't interfere with sleep. HEPA filters are also helpful in vacuum cleaners.
- Remove dust collectors (like books and magazines, where mold can grow) and, if possible, replace stuffed furniture with those made of "wipeable" surfaces such as wood, leather, or vinyl.
- When dusting, use a damp or treated cloth to avoid stirring up dust. After vacuuming, allow the dust to settle, then wipe surfaces down. Use a vacuum cleaner that contains the dust, rather than spewing it back out into the air.

Over time, intermittent breathing problems and periodic cutoff of oxygen (called hypoxemia) can stress the heart and lungs. Upper airway resistance syndrome is thought of as less severe than obstructive sleep apnea. However, UARS and sleep apnea are both associated with a greater risk of high blood pressure, cardiac arrhythmias, pulmonary hypertension, stroke, and, in severe cases, heart failure. In fact, a recent study in the *New England Journal of Medicine* found that even people with relatively mild sleep-disordered breathing had almost twice the risk of developing high blood pressure, compared to people with no breathing problems. In the Sleep Heart Health Study, we also found that the more apneas you have, the higher your risk.

Although obesity is a risk factor, thin women who have excess tissue in the soft palate and a narrow opening from the mouth to the pharynx area are also at high risk for upper airway resistance syndrome. Smoking is a risk factor for both sexes, as are drinking alcohol and using tranquilizers or muscle relaxants. The prevalence of snoring also increases as you get older, but you don't have to snore loudly (or at all) to have this syndrome.

Once diagnosed, treatments tend to be similar to those associated with apnea. Dental appliances and weight loss may correct the problem. For simple snoring, nasal sprays that reduce swelling can help, as can Breathe-Right and similar strips. They can actually increase nasal area by physically holding the nostrils open, and increasing muscle tone.

Obstructive Sleep Apnea

In obstructive sleep apnea, airflow to the lungs is briefly blocked in repeated episodes during the night. These episodes can last as long as a minute. And they can occur hundreds of times a night as you find yourself awakening and gasping for breath.

The blockage occurs somewhere between the nose or mouth and lungs. Most often it is in the throat. With each episode you make strong efforts to breathe and break the blockage in the airway. After many heaving attempts the blockage clears, usually with a loud snore or snort, and your breathing resumes normally. Unfortunately, to facilitate the clearing, your brain alerts and wakes up. In fact, it may be these awakenings that provide the muscle tone to clear the blockage. With each episode your oxygen level can decrease, and with each awakening your sleep is disturbed. In the morning you frequently feel tired, confused,

---

Factors Associated with Obstructive Sleep Apnea

- Increasing age
- Obesity
- Use of alcohol
- Use of sedating drugs
- Smoking
- Sleeping positions, especially sleeping on the back
- Hypothyroidism (underactive thyroid)
- Family history (other family members who snore and who have similar facial structure and dietary habits)
- Facial abnormalities
- Excessive airway tissue

---

and headachy. Your daytime energy is decreased, and you feel sleepy most of the day (this is often the only clue to obstructive sleep apnea). Sleep apnea may also be a cause of nocturia, or getting up frequently at night to urinate (this may be due to apnea's effects on urine excretion).

According to the National Sleep Foundation, as many as 18 million Americans have sleep apnea, twice as many men as women. But that may be an underestimate. We women may simply be outsnored by men (studies show that women are usually the ones who wake up and complain). Thanks to work by Dr. Terry Young, a professor of epidemiology at the University of Wisconsin, Madison, we know the disorder is not just a disease of overweight, aging men. Her work shows that women with apnea are probably misdiagnosed because of physician bias that apnea is a man's disease. Women have the same symptoms as men, but it is not clear if we are ever told so. When asked if they snore, most women say they don't know. It's possible our partners don't notice (because they're snoring away themselves or don't want to hurt our feelings). You may want to record your snoring, especially if you live alone, to be sure.

It's also true that we are somewhat protected by our estrogen and progesterone before menopause or if we are taking replacement estro-

Your Sleep Rx for Apnea

Besides the snore ball (see page 138), there are a number of treatments for obstructive sleep apnea, ranging from weight loss to surgery. In addition, we always warn patients to tell their treating physicians about the diagnosis to limit the use of sedating medications. Sedation (alcohol, too) can lengthen apneic events and increase the propensity to develop a full-blown attack of severe apnea.

Weight loss can be helpful, but, as we all know, it can be very difficult to lose weight if you're too sleepy to exercise and you've got a lot of weight to lose. It might help to know that sometimes you need to lose only a small amount of weight to correct the respiratory disorder.

One of the most effective apnea treatments is continuous positive airway pressure, or CPAP, a small air pump in a designer box. The air is pressurized to act as a pneumatic splint and keep the airway open during sleep. Air is piped through to your nose via a flexible hose connected to a small nasal mask, nasal prongs, or a full-face mask. Although it may not be sexy, the quiet, steady whisper of the pump is a big improvement over loud snores. Bed partners usually like it.

In fact, CPAP may have an added benefit in the bedroom. People with apnea frequently have decreased sex drive and compromised ability to achieve orgasm. A study of thirty men and women found that using a CPAP device resulted in improvement in both these areas. In fact, researchers at the national Naval Medical Center in Bethesda, Maryland, suggest that sleep apnea may be an unrecognized and reversible cause of sexual dysfunction.

The CPAP device is set for the correct level of air pressure after a night in the sleep lab. You use the device for each sleep period, then put it away for the day. You should feel better within days. We always encourage its use, if only for a brief time, so you'll have an awareness of how good you can feel with normal breathing during sleep. Then you can choose another treatment modality that's right for you.

We can also use adjustable mouth guards that extend the lower jaw, adding room to the airway. There are several varieties, and each needs to be individually fitted, possibly requiring several trips to the dentist. Be sure to find a practitioner with experience. The cost is about $1,500 and may not always be reimbursed by your insurance. Research indicates dental appliances can help with mild to moderate apnea.

Surgical solutions for apnea include tonsillectomies and adenoidectomies in children and the removal of any other floppy tissue in the throat or airway for adults. The most common surgery for apnea has been uvulopalatopharyngoplasty (UPPP), the cutting away of the uvula (that teardrop-shaped bit of flesh that hangs down in your throat), part of the soft palate, the tonsils, and possibly other excess tissue in the throat. This procedure typically requires general anesthesia and an overnight hospital stay. There's also an outpatient laser treatment (laser-assisted uvulopalatopharyngoplasty, or LAUP) to burn away the excess tissue, used for people with snoring and mild apnea. Both procedures are primarily effective for correcting problems related to the soft palate. It will be painful to swallow for about two weeks after the surgery. Laser procedures may be performed in repeated sessions until adequate control is gained. The surgery costs around $3,000, but it's reimbursed by most insurance plans if it's done to treat sleep apnea.

Somnoplasty is a new, virtually pain-free treatment for snoring and mild apnea. It shrinks soft tissue in the upper airway, including the base of the tongue, using radiofrequency energy. In this procedure a specially designed wand with an insulated needle electrode delivers low heat generated by radio waves to tissues beneath the mucus membrane, so there's no surface burn, dramatically reducing postoperative discomfort. The damaged tissues are naturally resorbed by the body in three to eight weeks, reducing excess tissue and opening the airway. Somnoplasty also scars and stiffens soft tissues, further shrinking them. Somnoplasty is done under local anesthesia on an outpatient basis and takes thirty to forty-five minutes in repeated visits. After the procedure you may experience some swelling and discomfort and need pain medications for two to three days. The cost is around $2,000, and, again, if it's done to treat breathing problems and sleep apnea, the procedure will be covered by insurance and Medicare.

The first long-term study of somnoplasty found that more than half the patients had no relapse in snoring for fourteen months after just one treatment. Other procedures using radiofrequency energy are being tested to cut tissues with less pain than conventional surgery.

You must decide on your treatment with your physician. It depends on your anatomy and the surgeon's experience. It is important to note that you should *always* have a follow-up sleep study to see whether your apnea has improved. Each form of surgery removes the area of the throat where the snoring sound occurs, so snoring will disappear, but the apnea may not. In fact, while most of these surgeries will cure snoring, they are only about 40 percent effective for curing apnea.

If you have low thyroid function (determined by a blood test) you may develop a form of apnea as well. Correcting the problem with replacement thyroid hormone may be all the help you need.

Because we know that sleep apnea may influence other diseases, such as hypertension and diabetes, it's very important to seek help if you (or your partner) snore, gasp during sleep, and are excessively sleepy in the daytime. The help you seek should begin with your own doctor, who can evaluate other illnesses through a complete physical including blood work. If necessary, you can be referred to a sleep center, where your sleep and breathing can be studied.

Remember, too, that even children can have significant apnea.

Large tonsils and adenoids are the usual culprits, and a tonsillectomy generally brings a complete cure. No one should tell you it doesn't matter if your child snores! Snoring is a signal that there is trouble in the airway, no matter who's snoring! I have seen children with severe oxygen deprivation from repetitive apneas through the night. No wonder they weren't growing and learning well!

gen. It seems that progesterone is a mild respiratory stimulant. In fact, a recent study of almost 2,000 women by the University of Toronto found that apnea is twice as likely to occur in postmenopausal women than in younger women, and is more severe when it does occur.

We know that body weight influences apnea. Fortunately, women are able to carry more weight than men without running into difficulty. A woman tends to carry excess weight in the hips and breasts (especially before menopause), whereas a man's extra pounds tend to end up on his belly or neck. Men have a larger waist-hip ratio (they're "apples," we're "pears"), which may be the culprit. That weight on the abdomen (such as with a late pregnancy) requires the lungs to suck harder to take in air. In the process the walls of the throat may be sucked closed and apnea may occur. Some studies suggest women have more hypopneas, partial apneas. When women do have apneas, they may be shorter than those experienced by men. This may have to do with the anatomy of the upper airway or other female physiology. A number of researchers report that women with sleep apnea take longer to fall asleep and have more slow-wave sleep and fewer nighttime awakenings than men (but that may be more related to our female sleep patterns).

At equal weight, a man would probably have more sleep apnea than a woman would. However, a woman who has very large and heavy breasts may be at risk because the weight of the breast tissue may affect her ability to move her rib cage and breathe. Also, women who are severely overweight are in jeopardy at any age. They may not have apnea from airway obstruction but may make less effort to breathe in REM

Treatments for Obstructive Sleep Apnea

- Weight loss
- Repositioning (snore ball)
- Behavioral changes, such as stopping alcohol and tobacco use
- Continuous positive airway pressure device (CPAP)
- Surgeries:
  Tonsillectomy
  Uvulopalatopharyngoplasty (UPPP)
  Laser-assisted uvulopalatopharyngoplasty (LAUP)
  Somnoplasty
- Dental appliance
- Thyroid hormone replacement

---

sleep, thereby depriving themselves of enough oxygen. This is called hypoventilation of obesity. We have seen a number of such women in our laboratory. Their treatment is similar to but sometimes more complicated than the treatment for apnea alone.

Sleep apnea can also be caused by the position in which you sleep. When some people sleep on their backs, gravity pulls excess airway tissues down into the throat. You'll recognize this one. Your partner only snores, or snores more loudly, on his or her back. A nudge (or a kick in the shins) prompts the person to roll over, and the noise lessens or ceases. In these cases we often recommend making a snore ball, cutting a tennis ball in half and sewing it into a pocket in a tight-fitting T-shirt with the cut side down. The snorer wears the T-shirt backward (with the pocket and ball on the back), so that when the sleeper rolls over onto his or her back, the bulk of the ball encourages him or her to roll right back over again, decreasing snoring and apneic episodes. It's a very low-tech solution, but it helps positional sleep apnea.

Pregnancy and Apnea

Women can develop a temporary form of sleep apnea during pregnancy, because the girth of the abdomen, causing constriction of the diaphragm, leads to breathing problems. I have seen some significant apnea develop among already obese women who are pregnant. In those cases both the women and presumably the fetuses suffered severe oxygen loss intermittently through the night. This could lead to increased risk to the mother's health, as well as to the fetus's.

In fact, a recent study of five hundred Swedish women found that habitual snoring was a sign of pregnancy-induced high blood pressure (preeclampsia) and was associated with lower birth weights and lower Apgar scores (an evaluation of a newborn's heart rate, respiratory effort, muscle tone, response to stimulation, and skin color). The study also noted that women started to snore before any sign of preeclampsia appeared and that the snoring was related to sleep apnea. So if you're snoring during the later months of your pregnancy, mention it to your doctor. It is easy to monitor oxygen levels during the night at home. That would be a first step to see how much the snoring (and maybe apnea) is affecting your pregnancy. (Preeclampsia can be a serious problem. When placental blood flow is hampered by hypertension, it can starve the fetus of oxygen and cause low birth weight and even stillbirth. Signs of preeclampsia include sudden, rapid weight gain and fluid retention.)

You could also make a tape of the snoring. Set a recorder by the bed—make sure, of course, that you're recording *your* snoring, not your partner's! If you hear gasping and snorting as well, you may need a sleep study to determine the correct treatment until delivery. An immediate help is to sleep in a recliner. That way, the baby isn't pressing so heavily on your diaphragm and you'll breathe more easily.

Narcolepsy: Sleep Attacks

Narcolepsy is a lifelong central nervous system disorder marked by uncontrollable urges to sleep during waking hours. In fact, people with narcolepsy have difficulty staying asleep at night and staying awake during the day. It is almost as though they cannot stay in any one state of consciousness, waking, NREM sleep, or REM sleep.

Many times you'll see jokes about people falling asleep at the dinner table with their faces in the food. Believe me, narcolepsy is no joke. Frequently, people with symptoms consult five to seven clinicians before they get a correct diagnosis. That journey may take ten to fifteen years! Think about being misunderstood and pathologically sleepy all those years. Think about how it could affect your lifestyle if it began in your teen years. Everyone calls you lazy or stupid, and you can't stay awake. Neither can you learn or develop to your full potential. This disorder affects about one in every two thousand American men and women. As far as we know, narcolepsy is an equal opportunity disorder. It hits as many men as women. And *hit* may be the correct term. Narcolepsy tends to arrive in the second decade of life, although we now note many younger children with the disorder. We are not entirely sure about the cause, but research is moving very quickly. In some cases there is a genetic component. In others we suspect some illness or emotional trigger. Perhaps there is a combination of causes.

Fortunately, there is a narcoleptic dog colony at Stanford University under the direction of Dr. Emanuel Mignot, which provides a wonderful opportunity to study the disorder. Now, for many of you the thought of research on animals may be distasteful. However, because of these dogs, researchers have just found a gene that is responsible for symptoms of narcolepsy. It's called the *hypocretin receptor 2 gene.* The gene encodes for a protein on the surface of brain cells that functions as a kind of antenna, allowing the cells to receive messages from other cells, including those that promote wakefulness. When the gene is defective, the cells can't receive these messages. As a result, the dogs suffer sleep attacks.

About the same time researchers in Texas were able to develop a mouse without this gene and also saw symptoms of narcolepsy. It's very likely that the same gene in humans contributes to this disorder. In early 2000 researchers from California and the Netherlands reported that underexpression of the neural protein hypocretin-1 may be a cause of narcolepsy in humans. This groundbreaking work will undoubtedly provide better treatments and, perhaps, eventual cure of this disorder.

Narcolepsy is not your usual sleepiness. There are six key symptoms

Drugs Used to Treat Narcolepsy

Brand Name	Generic Name	Dose (mg/day)
FOR WAKEFULNESS		
Provigil	modafinil	200–800
Ritalin	methylphenidate	5–100
Dexedrine	dextroamphetamine/	5–100
	methamphetamine	
Cylert*	pemoline	37.5–300
FOR CATAPLEXY		
Vivactil	protriptyline	10–60
Prozac	fluoxetine	20–80

*Cylert has recently been linked to fatal liver toxicity and may not be your best choice.

of narcolepsy: profound and excessive daytime sleepiness, cataplexy, sleep paralysis, hypnagogic sleep-like hallucinations, automatic behavior, and fragmented nighttime sleep. Not all symptoms need be present to make a diagnosis of the disorder, and not all symptoms develop at the same time or ever. Some people will develop cataplexy after several years of sleepiness but may never have sleep paralysis. Cataplexy is thought to be a brief intrusion of REM sleep, or at least a part of REM sleep, into our state of wakefulness. In Chapter 1, I mentioned that we are paralyzed in REM sleep. Cataplexy is a carryover of that paralysis and is triggered by emotional situations. The major trigger is laughter, of all things, with anger or excitement being a close second.

The symptom of paralysis may be mild, the weakening of a facial muscle or a bob of the head, or it could be total collapse to the ground. During the few seconds of the event, the person is awake, able to see and hear, but unable to move. When it's over she regains her muscle tone (strength) and carries on as before, maybe embarrassed but fine. As you can imagine, cataplexy can spill over into many aspects of one's life. It can happen in public or private. One of the most difficult times is during the excitement of sexual activity. Imagine becoming suddenly paralyzed during sex! Many people find the best way to treat the symptom is to avoid the triggering events. That's hard on everyone. What would your life be without laughter and sexual excitement?

One of my most memorable narcoleptic patients was a woman of fifty-five who had been symptomatic since her teen years! She'd used stimulant medication in the form of diet pills for more than thirty years. The pills kept her awake. She also opened her own shop and was able to nap in the back. This was a woman of extreme drive and forbearance who made the best of her life. She also had severe cataplexy and a wicked sense of humor. We all had to watch out when she told a joke, because she (and her two hundred pounds) would fall.

An African American woman once told me that the symptoms of narcolepsy were called the black woman's disease. She informed me that many black women have a "sleeping disease" (including sleep paralysis). In my experience and that of some other sleep researchers, the symptom of cataplexy appears to be expressed differently in African Americans. Rather than have a muscle collapse or weakness, they tend to suddenly fall asleep in the same emotional setting that would cause full-blown cataplexy in others. The angry mother of a young male patient told me she would get annoyed with him because every time she yelled at him he would fall asleep, even standing. She thought he was being disrespectful! You can see that narcolepsy can cause misunderstandings even among those you love.

Narcolepsy may cause hypnagogic hallucinations, usually visual, when a person is fighting off a sleep attack. For instance, someone may "see" a tree in the middle of a highway and slam on the car brakes. Others describe "seeing" people in their bedroom. This is probably an intrusion of REM sleep into the waking state. It can also cause automatic behavior, such as forgetting something on the stove or driving past your destination.

Sleep paralysis is a similar intrusion of REM sleep. But this time it occurs upon awakening. You wake up but find that you cannot move, that you couldn't answer the phone or run if a fire alarm rang. For someone with narcolepsy, this is very frightening! Even though people understand it, fright is part of the event. A quick cure is tactile contact. If another person touches your arm, the paralysis breaks. You can also try to cure the paralysis yourself by moving the two muscles that function in REM sleep: the eye muscles and the diaphragm. So attempting to take a deep breath or moving the eyes rapidly is helpful. If you suspect symptoms of narcolepsy, a sleep disorder center is your best source of diagnosis and treatment. Narcolepsy is diagnosed by polysomnogram (a sleep study) and daytime testing of naps. The treatment is medication to increase wakefulness and to reduce cataplexy and symptoms of REM sleep. In the past only stimulant medications were available to increase wakefulness. Now the drug modafinil (Provigil) enhances wakefulness. It's a vast improvement over older stimulants, which could be habit-forming. Antidepressants that retard REM sleep are used to control cataplexy.

At the New York University Sleep Disorders Center, we were part of the multicenter studies in which Provigil was evaluated. There were few side effects and no rush or crash, which is most common with stimulant medications. That is probably because Provigil is a novel wake promoter, not a stimulant. It works differently in the brain. It is also long-lasting, so you only need to take it once a day. It has a very low abuse potential and does not develop tolerance. Since it is not classified as a medication that can lead to dependency, modafinil does not require special prescriptions or frequent appointments for renewals.

People who suffer from sleepiness from other causes and must drive or are in a sensitive occupation might consider modafinil to help maintain wakefulness and keep safe on the road. For more information, see the chart on page 141. Along with medications, social support and education are valuable additions to care. There are a number of support groups listed in Appendix II.

Isolated Sleep Paralysis

Another form of sleep paralysis occurs in the absence of a sleep disorder; it's called isolated sleep paralysis. It's believed to affect 40 to 50 percent of people at least once in their lives and has been described since ancient times, across many cultures, and by many names.

The sensations of fright and constriction in the chest that accompany sleep paralysis are often described as a witch or ghost that sits on the sleeper's chest. African American tradition (with and without narcolepsy) calls it "being ridden by the witch" or the "witch riding on your chest." The Chinese call it "ghost pressure" (*gui ya*); people in the West Indies call it *kokma,* a ghost baby who jumps on a sleeper's chest.

In isolated sleep paralysis, the brain and body seem disconnected, as though you're on the edge of sleep. As I mentioned, this is the same paralysis that occurs during REM sleep. But it happens when you're just emerging from sleep. You experience the sensation of being awake while dreaming and you cannot move. After a few moments the brain and body resume communication, and you can move again. This can be a frightening experience. But if it occurs without other symptoms, especially those of narcolepsy, it's really nothing to worry about. Check with your doctor.

Restless Legs Syndrome and Periodic Leg Movements

Restless legs syndrome chronically affects about 5–10 percent of the adult population. It is best described as a compelling urge to move accompanied by "creepy-crawly" sensations in your legs. Some patients say it feel like Pepsi-Cola in the veins. The feeling can also occur in your arms.

The sensations begin around bedtime, having a circadian rhythm of their own. The sensations start or are made worse by rest. To get relief you need to move, run, rub, or walk. You can imagine how that would interfere with sleep. In fact, the sensations prevent sleep in many cases or disturb it for an hour or two. As I discussed earlier, they also seem to affect women during pregnancy.

A related disorder is periodic leg movements, jerking rhythmic movements, most of which occur in the legs every twenty to forty seconds across the night, disrupting sleep. Each time the leg muscles twitch, brain changes, including wakefulness, occur. This is not the same as those leg cramps or twitches that happen at sleep onset. Restless legs, and to some extent periodic leg movements, have also been associated with diabetic peripheral neuropathy, vascular illnesses, kidney disease, and iron deficiency anemia. Good control of the underlying condition

Your Sleep Rx for Restless Legs

Drugs which increase or substitute for the neurotransmitter dopamine, which affects movement, can be very useful in treating restless legs. Many of these are the same drugs used to treat Parkinson's disease, but the doses are generally much smaller. They include: carbidopa/LevoDopa, Sinemet, pergolide (Permax), pramipexole (Mirapex), bromocriptine (Parlodel), selegiline (Eldepryl), and ropinirole (Requip). Opiate medications commonly used to reduce pain also provide some benefit, although the doses needed are usually higher than those required for pain relief. These medications include: propoxyphene (Darvocet), codeine, Tylenol #3 with oxycodone (Percocet), hydrocodone (Vicodin), and pentazocine (Talwin). Several of these compounds are combined with acetaminophen or aspirin, and the dose has to be carefully watched to avoid side effects of these products. Other treatments have been used with varying effects. These include hypnotic and sedative medications to blunt the brain's alerting response to the activity like triazolam (Halcion), clonazepam (Klonopin), alprazolam (Xanax), diazepam (Valium), zaleplon (Sonata), temazepam (Restoril), and zolpidem (Ambien).

In addition, antiseizure medications such as gabapentin (Neurontin), carbamazepine (Tegretol), and valproic acid (Depakote) have been used successfully for restless legs syndrome. Other classes of drugs—including antidepressants (although they can make things worse in some cases) such as the SSRI fluoxetine (Prozac) or the tricyclic imipramine (Tofranil); Lioresal (baclofen), also used in multiple sclerosis; and antihypertension medications such as clonidine (Catapres) and propranolol (Inderal)—can also be effective. Of these, Neurontin is perhaps the most commonly used and one with the fewest side effects, especially in the elderly.

Your choice of medication must be made with your physician, based on other medications you may be taking or other illnesses you have. Along with medications, behavioral treatments such as relaxation therapy, massage, biofeedback, or the trick of keeping your mind active with challenging games or work will help. Avoiding alcohol can also help.

We're fortunate that some state-of-the-art research is being done by Drs. Richard Allen and Christopher Earley at Johns Hopkins in Baltimore, Maryland, and Arthur Walters and Wayne Henning at the JFK Memorial Medical Center in Edison, New Jersey, to establish the cause of this disorder. The Hopkins scientists have shown that the sensations may be linked to an insufficiency of brain iron. Even though iron levels in the blood may be normal, the level of tissue content of iron in the brain may be low. So increasing oral iron intake could be helpful.

Iron supplements can be taken along with vitamin C to aid absorption. But, please, don't start taking iron supplements without consulting your physician! There are side effects, such as constipation, and interactions with drugs like Coumadin; in rare cases, iron overdose can be fatal. Ask your doctor about taking vitamin B12 and folic acid, which may also help restless legs.

will help relieve symptoms. You should know that in women particularly, alcohol worsens the situation, as can tricyclic antidepressants.

Nocturnal Eating Disorder

Can you imagine going into your kitchen in the morning to find that someone ate all your groceries in the night . . . and it was you? Women with nocturnal eating disorder may do this every night. It's considered a parasomnia similar to sleepwalking.

In this disorder women rise suddenly while sleeping or when partially asleep and eat anything and everything in the refrigerator (50 percent of them have been shown to be asleep!). Many patients report feeling half awake, half asleep during episodes and describe their eating

Medications Used for Restless Legs

Generic Name	Brand Name	Dose
ANTI-PARKINSON DRUGS		
levodopa	Sinemet	25/100 mg to start; may be repeated once during the night
pergolide	Permax	½ tablet of 0.05 mg to start 0.5 mg–0.75 mg/day
pramipexole	Mirapex	0.125–1.0 mg/day
bromocriptine	Parlodel	5–15 mg/day
rapinirole	Requip	0.5–12 mg/day
HYPNOTICS/SEDATIVES		
triazolam	Halcion	0.125–0.25 mg/day
alprazolam	Xanax	0.25–2 mg/day
clonazepam	Klonopin	0.5–2 mg/day
diazepam	Valium	5–10 mg/day
PAIN MEDICATIONS		
propoxyphene	Darvon	3–4 tabs/day
hydrocodone	Vicodin	5–40 mg/day
oxycodone	Percodan	5–40 mg/day
ANTISEIZURE DRUGS		
gabapentin	Neurontin	300–900 mg at time of sleep
carbamazepine	Tegretol	100–300 mg/day
divalproex (valproic acid)	Depakote	125–500 mg/day
ANTIHYPERTENSIVES		
clonidine	Catapres	0.1–0.3 mg at time of sleep
propranolol	Inderal	5–10 mg at time of sleep
ANTIDEPRESSANTS (USE WITH CAUTION, AS THEY MAY INCREASE THE PROBLEM)		
fluoxetine	Prozac	varies
imipramine	Tofranil	varies
trazodone	Desyrel	varies

as binge eating. The behavior continues compulsively even if the patient "wakes" up. An odd assortment of foods are eaten with abandon, raw or frozen food may be eaten, and patients may even engage in complicated cooking procedures.

Most patients initially deny any awareness of their nighttime eating, but they cannot contradict the effect: kitchen messes in the morning and obesity. Two internationally known sleep clinicians and researchers from the University of Minnesota, Carlos H. Schenck and Mark W. Mahawold, found that patients with nocturnal eating disorder never report being thirsty or hungry at night, and they have no indigestion or feelings of fullness after eating episodes. They rarely drink alcohol or smoke during their nighttime eating episodes. They seem to prefer thick liquids and foods (like soup). Episodes can occur during the week, on weekends, even on vacation. A recent study found that patients begin having sleep disturbances around age fifteen, with eating-related episodes starting in the mid- to late twenties. Some patients may eat as many as six times during the night.

This disorder occurs more frequently in women, and it seems to be related to increased daytime stress (although that's not the only cause). A common stressor is a history of physical abuse or other concerns about safety at night. One study found that as many as 70 percent of patients had other sleep disorders, such as sleepwalking, restless legs syndrome, and apnea, which contributed to their arousals. The phenomenon can be associated with other eating disorders, such as bulimia, binge eating disorder, or anorexia nervosa, as well as chronic dieting. Many patients report taking psychiatric medications, such as benzodiazepines, antidepressants, and antipsychotics (which may have influenced their symptoms as well).

Besides the obvious health problem of obesity, this habit has dangerous consequences if a woman eats food that is spoiled, raw, or to which she is allergic, or that will interact with medications she may be taking (for example, cheese with antidepressants called MAO inhibitors), or even nonfood items that may be toxic (one study reported that a patient drank fingernail polish).

For that reason, it's always important to tell your doctor if you think you've been eating in the middle of the night. An added safety problem is the possibility that you will return to bed having left the stove or other cooking equipment on.

A number of treatment strategies for nocturnal eating disorder have been tried. The successful ones include treatment of any underlying causes of sleep arousal and underlying stressors. In addition, behavioral reinforcement sometimes works. There have been interesting reports of success with strong reinforcement reward therapies. For instance, a woman gave all her jewelry to the therapist and would get a piece back each time she didn't eat during the night! Medications such as fluoxetine (Prozac) or clonazepam (Klonopin) are often helpful. Fluoxetine may reduce the compulsive nature of the problem, and clonazepam decreases one's ability to awaken and move during sleep, so it may prevent the episode just as it may other sleepwalking events.

Night Eating Syndrome

We've all had the occasional attack of the munchies at night. But this problem is quite different. It is also different from nocturnal eating disorder because people with night eating syndrome are awake.

In night eating syndrome, people engage in rapid binge eating late at night, have difficulty falling asleep until way after midnight, awaken (sometimes repeatedly) during the night and eat again, then eat little or nothing early in the day. In fact, some take in as many as 56 percent of their calories at night.

Individuals are fully alert during each episode; they have no amnesia about their nighttime eating. This disorder is said to affect about 1.5 percent of the general population, perhaps as many as 10 percent of obese people seeking treatment for their weight.

Disruptions in circadian rhythms and in hormones related to sleep, hunger, and stress may play a role in this disorder. In a 1999 report in the *Journal of the American Medical Association,* researchers at the University Hospital in Trømso, Norway, found that people with the disorder did not have the normal increase in the hormones melatonin (which induces and maintains sleep) and leptin (which controls appetite and has been linked to obesity), while they experienced elevations of the stress hormone cortisol over a twenty-four-hour period.

In the same report, the pattern of behavior in patients observed by Dr. Albert Stunkard, director of the Weight and Eating Disorders Program at the University of Pennsylvania, started out as morning "anorexia," eating nothing at all during the morning and taking in fewer than average calories during the day, with increasing depression. At night patients' mood worsened, and they raided the kitchen for mostly high-carbohydrate snacks (which elevate levels of serotonin in the brain, helping to boost mood and promoting sleep). The cycle of increased depression and anxiety with bouts of binge eating continues through the night. Dr. Stunkard speculates that this eating pattern may be a way to self-medicate an underlying stress response that leads to disturbed sleep in vulnerable people.

This is a newly identified eating disorder, so more research needs to be done on it. But it's important to alert your doctor. It's possible that taking melatonin may help, as may antidepressants called SSRIs (selective serotonin reuptake inhibitors like Prozac or Paxil), which raise levels of serotonin in the brain. Since this disorder (and nocturnal eating disorder) also appears to be related to stress, stress reduction measures (see pages 30–31) may also be beneficial.

Real Nightmares: Post-Traumatic Stress Disorder

Women who have been victims of violence may experience sleep disruptions, or post-traumatic stress disorder (PTSD), which can produce vivid nightmares (and waking flashbacks) of the abuse.

Barbara was a young woman in her early twenties who had begun to experience sleep difficulty that was clearly tied to a significant and unpleasant incident. She was home alone when she was injured by an intruder and from that moment had become very fearful about being alone. Immediately after this event Barbara had gone to her parents' home and was able to sleep well. But when she returned to her own apartment, she had trouble sleeping again. It was clear that no matter how often she dealt with the incident in my consultations with her, the memory was so vivid that there was no way for her to relax and sleep. She had tried numerous sleeping medications and antidepressant drugs, and had been in therapy. But she was still reliving the incident in her mind and experienced vivid nightmares and flashbacks.

Barbara was suffering from PTSD. I suggested that she utilize a new technique called Eye Movement Desensitization Reprocessing (EMDR). This technique helps restructure thinking about a traumatic event while using a specific form of bilateral stimulation. The patient is asked to recall the incident, to think of the bad feelings associated with it, to name them, and then to think about how she would like to change the way she viewed the event. For Barbara, feelings of helplessness and isolation permeated her memories of the incident. She chose a positive view that she was strong and competent to care for herself.

During an EMDR session, the patient is asked to move her eyes from side to side very rapidly, have her hands or legs tapped in an alternating (left, right, left, right) pattern, or listen to sounds alternating in her left and right ears. While this is going on, the patient visualizes the event and her cognition about it. This is a controversial procedure, best carried out with a specially trained mental health professional. Barbara had great success with EMDR and found that she was able to remove the negative thoughts from her mind and relax enough to begin to go back to normal sleep patterns.

What I see in women who have undergone traumatic events and found their way to the sleep center is that stress seems to be a huge factor in their ability to sleep. For some women, a pivotal occasion (but not necessarily a traumatic event, such as an assault) sets a pattern of anxiety in motion, and over the years that pattern takes on a life of its own. By the time I see these women, I must act as a detective, tracking the pattern to see when it began and how we can change the habits that have perpetuated it.

Parasomnias

Parasomnias are defined as physical problems that occur around sleep (*para* means "around," *somnia* means "sleep"). They include sleepwalking and night terrors, which occur most often when a person is half-aroused or aroused from sleep, and nightmares and sleep paralysis, which are associated with REM sleep and the transition to other sleep stages. Parasomnias do not affect the processes actually responsible for sleep and awake states, but they do reflect activation of the central nervous system around sleep.

Rayanne was a young woman who came to the center reporting some unusual "dream or nightmare/terror" activity. She remembered "waking" to see her husband being attacked. She went to his "rescue" only to wind up punching her husband (thinking he was the aggressor) and injuring him. Such events had happened since her childhood. She would wake to "see things" she recognized were not true, then roll over and return to sleep. In the weeks before she consulted me, however, she had been under increasing stress.

Rayanne's striking her husband was particularly vivid, and she acted out before realizing what was happening. In talking with her, it became clear to me that she had hit her husband not in a dream state but rather while coming out of a state of slow-wave or very deep sleep. She was having a confusional arousal.

This experience is common in children as they progress from slow-wave sleep into a lighter state of sleep. They may sleepwalk, talk, or wet the bed. There is a vast difference between dreaming and having a confusional arousal. During a confusional arousal, the person is not paralyzed as in REM sleep and can act out thoughts, or even routine complex activities. Some people have driven in this state or committed violent acts.

Rayanne had been a sleepwalker and a sleep talker as a child. Her parasomnias seemed worse when she was stressed or sleep-deprived. This is all very typical. The issue is what to do about them.

The first step was to help Rayanne understand the mechanics of the problem and realize that it wasn't something she could control. This was very helpful to her. Rayanne also had to address her stress level and find ways to relax before sleep. In addition she was instructed to avoid sleep deprivation because it would deepen her sleep and hence the potential for parasomnias. But she still suffered from them, with the potential to hurt herself, her husband, or anyone else who was in her way at the time. We eventually prescribed medication to reduce Rayanne's arousals from sleep and suggested some behavioral interventions she could use to aid her safety, especially when she traveled.

The difference between nightmares and night terrors is timing. In

Your Sleep Rx for Parasomnias

If you suffer from parasomnias, maintain good sleep habits and use my tips for stabilizing your sleep system (see pages 21–26) so you don't become sleep-deprived. This includes avoiding vigorous exercise too close to bedtime, which we know can deepen slow-wave sleep.

Try to lighten deep sleep by leaving a light on in the room or having some soft music playing. I think everyone can relate to the fact that you don't seem to sleep as deeply when there is background noise.

Find ways to build a safe environment, such as removing throw rugs and pushing furniture back against the walls. I suggest to adult patients that they buy an electric eye device used to detect intruders. They can put the electric eye across the room's entrance and exit so that noise will awaken them if they get out of bed.

In some cases medications and stress reduction can help. A drug such as the benzodiazepine clonazepam (Klonopin) increases atonia and lightens the depth of the delta sleep. It's also a good muscle relaxant, which may limit the ability to move and get up during these incomplete arousals. Stress reduction can help reduce arousals from sleep as well.

For bruxism, your dentist can make a tooth guard that will reduce wear and tear on your teeth. Stress reduction may lessen the number of events.

Frontal lobe epilepsy should be treated with antiepileptic drugs such as divalproex (Depakote) or carbamazepine (Tegretol). These will lessen or completely control the event.

nightmares the person is in REM sleep. She experiences the nightmare every seventy to ninety minutes across the night and may remember a story line to her dream. In night terrors she is emerging from short-wave sleep soon after sleep began. She therefore has no awareness of a bad dream or memory of the event later. Her reaction is the aftermath of

panic, terror, violence, and aggression. She may get up and attack someone or display "fight or flight" behavior if awakened. My colleague Dr.
Rosalind Cartwright, director of the Sleep Disorder Service and
Research Center at Rush–Presbyterian–St. Luke's Medical Center in
Chicago, suggests that night terrors evoke a strong self-preservation
drive. She notes that terrors are different physiologically from dreaming;
the chemistry and psychology are different, too.

Other types of parasomnias include teeth grinding (bruxism) and
nocturnal paroxysmal dystonia, now felt to be frontal lobe epilepsy. In
frontal lobe epilepsy, people scream and throw themselves out of bed,
frequently injuring themselves. They also make stereotypic movements
like pedaling a bicycle while in bed. These events may occur several
times across the night.

When You're in Pain

Unfortunately, more women than men develop painful connective
tissue disorders and autoimmune diseases, and frequently these disorders are exacerbated by hormonal fluctuations and sometimes by
menopause. Among the disorders that disrupt sleep are fibromyalgia,
lupus, multiple sclerosis, and rheumatoid arthritis.

Some disorders, like lupus, affect a variety of organs and nerve tissue. Others, such as multiple sclerosis, affect the nerve fibers leading to
and from skeletal muscles. Some diseases, like multiple sclerosis, are
cyclic, going into remission for months or years, then flaring up under
stress.

Within the sleep world fibromyalgia is the most well-studied condition in this category. We know, for instance, that women with this
disease may show a specific type of brain wave that looks like wake in
sleep. Curiously, 15 percent of healthy people have this pattern and do
not complain about poor sleep. This pattern has also been noted among
people with depression. Women with fibromyalgia frequently complain
of nonrefreshing sleep and daytime sleepiness. Studies show that disruptions in slow-wave sleep may lower the threshold for musculoskeletal
pain in middle-aged women and may be a factor in fibromyalgia.

A number of treatments for fibromyalgia have been tried. One is medication. Low-dose tricyclic antidepressants at bedtime can help the patient feel more rested but do nothing for the brain-wave pattern. We also know that late-afternoon aerobic exercise will deepen sleep and prevent fibromyalgia. Frequently the disorder is seen in combination with depression. Again, it is very hard to say which comes first, but treating the depression may clear up the sleep disruption.

For arthritis or muscle pain, an analgesic designed for nighttime use, like acetaminophen with diphenhydramine (Tylenol PM and generics), can help relieve pain and promote sleep. New nonsteroidal, anti-inflammatory medications (NSAIDs) that do not cause as many gastrointestinal problems as aspirin can also be effective pain relievers. Among these are refecoxib (Vioxx) and celecoxib (Celebrex). On occasion, cortisone may be needed. This can be very disruptive to sleep, causing insomnia and vivid dreams.

Other methods for reducing pain and increasing sleep-promoting relaxation include biofeedback, meditation, and yoga. And don't forget those hot baths, which not only soothe joint pain but help you sleep better.

Headaches and Sleep

Headaches, mostly migraines and tension-type headaches, are another "female" problem frequently experienced during sleep or when one is just waking.

Some 23 million women suffer from migraine headaches, outnumbering male sufferers three to one. Some migraines may be related to hormones, with a falling estrogen level thought to be a powerful trigger. So women may experience migraines when estrogen dips premenstrually or during pill-free days if they're taking oral contraceptives. (Other women may find that oral contraceptives worsen migraines.) Pregnancy may either lessen or bring out migraines. Migraines may surface for the first time (or reappear after an initial episode in the teens or early twenties) in perimenopausal women, and women who've had occasional migraines may have more of them as they pass through menopause.

Migraine headaches are often felt on one side of the head or behind one eye, but the pain can often migrate to the other side. In a "classic

Your Sleep Rx for Headaches

An important treatment for headaches is to prevent sleep loss and maintain good sleep hygiene (those Four Rs again). Falling asleep on couches and planes could well indicate the need for more nocturnal sleep! It is also helpful for you and your doctor to remember that most effective headache medications will have an effect on sleep, either good or bad. Be alert to interactions and use medications for their benefits.

A number of medications can prevent or abort migraine headaches. The most effective are the triptan medications, such as sumatriptan (Imitrex), naratriptan (Amerge), rizatriptan (Maxalt), and zolmitriptan (Zomig). These drugs attach to receptors for 5-hydroxytryptamine (5-HT, a precursor of serotonin) and mimic its action, stopping inflammation around nerves and blood vessels, and constricting dilated blood vessels. They also reduce the nausea and light sensitivity that often accompany a migraine. Side effects can include constriction of the throat or chest, so such drugs should not be used by women with coronary heart disease, ischemic heart disease (restricted blood flow to the heart), or uncontrolled high blood pressure, or women who are pregnant.

Ergotamine tartrate preparations, such as Cafergot and Wigraine (or a drug put under the tongue, Ergostat), also act on 5-HT receptors.

Some migraines may respond to antidepressants, particularly SSRIs, fluoxetine (Prozac) and its relatives, which prevent serotonin from being reabsorbed by brain cells and thereby keep serotonin levels higher. However, some of these medications can cause insomnia. If your physician recommends you take a dosage at bedtime, paroxetine (Paxil) could be a better choice, since it seems to be less stimulating.

Menstrual migraines may respond to estrogen in oral or patch form. Women taking oral contraceptives who find they have migraines during pill-free days can, under careful supervision by a physician, take the pill on a continuous basis, with "withdrawal bleeding" every few months. You can also try to prevent menstrual migraines by taking a drug such as naproxen sodium (Anaprox), naproxen (Naprosyn), prescription-strength ibuprofen (Motrin), or a double dose of over-the-counter strength (220 milligrams) naproxen sodium two days before your period and continuing through your menstrual flow. These nonsteroidal, anti-inflammatory drugs (NSAIDs) may keep blood vessels from dilating by inhibiting production of prostaglandins. However, this should be done only under a physician's supervision.

The herb feverfew has been shown to be an effective migraine preventive and reliever (it may also help with cluster and menstrual headaches). Feverfew contains compounds that inhibit inflammation, improve blood vessel tone, and affect serotonin. The generally accepted dose is 125 milligrams of prepared, dried feverfew (containing at least 0.2 percent of the active ingredient parthenolide). Side effects of feverfew can include mouth sores and stomach upset. (For more on herbal products, see page 75.) Biofeedback has also been successful in treating migraines.

Treatments for cluster headaches include drugs containing ergotamine, sumatriptan, antidepressants like amitriptyline (which interferes with pain signals from the brain), steroids like prednisone (which reduce inflammation), and even inhaling oxygen for ten to fifteen minutes, since blood oxygen levels have been found to be lower during a cluster attack.

Drugs used for migraines can also help tension headaches. Massage of the neck area is useful, and drugs like ibuprofen can help to reduce pain and muscle tension in less severe cases. One of the specific treatments for paroxysmal nocturnal headache is indomethacin (Indocin) in doses of 50 milligrams taken at night.

However, daily use of headache medications can cause rebound headaches, which occur when the body has become so dependent on the medication that when it wears off the pain starts up again, prompting another dose. This cycle may only be halted by stopping the medications for a time.

Some researchers advocate taking extra magnesium as a way to prevent migraine (and perhaps cluster) headaches. Magnesium is believed to play a role in regulating blood vessel tone and serotonin function. One study estimated that 50 percent of migraine sufferers were deficient in magnesium. Taking 600 milligrams of slow-release magnesium (Slow-Mag) may help, as will making sure you have enough magnesium in your diet (from foods like legumes, dark, leafy vegetables, seafood, and whole grains; see the box on page 58).

Headache clinics often advise people to avoid headache-inducing foods. These include anything with the preservative nitrate, such as lunch meats and wine, and foods containing monosodium glutamate (MSG).

migraine," a woman may see an aura, typically zigzag lights that start out small but may eventually fill the field of vision; headaches may appear shortly after the aura. This phenomenon affects 10 to 15 percent of people with migraines. Most women experience migraines without aura (a few may have just the visual aura, called an ocular migraine). A woman may also have nausea and light sensitivity during a migraine and find that movement makes her symptoms worse. Migraines can be extremely disabling, lasting from two to seventy-two hours. Some people find lying down in a dark room and sleeping (along with medication) can help get rid of a migraine.

It seems strange that migraine headaches could be caused by sleep when so many people find they are relieved by sleep. However, people with parasomnias tend to have more migraines. One link may be the neurotransmitter serotonin, which is involved in regulating sleep, experiencing pain, and even triggering depression. When levels of serotonin are low, we tend to see more migraines. Serotonin is also known to constrict blood vessels; when serotonin levels are low, the vessels may dilate, sending blood pulsing through too-full vessels and causing the pounding sensation of a migraine. That's why treatment is built around triptan drugs like sumatriptan (Imitrex), which react with specific serotonin receptors in the brain, or the antidepressants called SSRIs, which increase serotonin levels.

Tension-type headaches can be triggered by stress but may also be related to muscle spasms in the head and neck (some people may have accompanying pain in the shoulders and neck). The pain usually begins in the muscles at the back of the head, working its way up to the forehead or temples. Most people describe the headaches as feeling as if their head were caught in a vise. Many experts believe these headaches, although related to muscle pain, are caused by the same biochemical process that leads to migraines. In fact, many women with migraines also have chronic tension-type headaches.

How can tension headaches be related to sleep, when during sleep we should be totally relaxed? Stress can take its toll in chronic muscle contraction, which can irritate nerves and contractile muscle fibers. As a result, pain may linger long after our muscles have relaxed. This is why we may wake up on Saturday after a stressful week with a tension headache.

Cluster headaches, which *are* a nighttime problem, are far are less common in women (85 percent of sufferers are men). These headaches usually arise between 9:00 P.M. and 10:00 A.M.; around 75 percent occur during sleep itself, usually during REM sleep. They also appear to be linked to our circadian rhythm (and its effect on the vascular system), sometimes occurring daily for two weeks. A good clue to a cluster headache is the timing of the pain. Remember, REM sleep cycles through the night every seventy to ninety minutes. The cycles get longer toward morning, and the longest one may be twenty minutes or more. If you're waking with a headache toward morning, chances are it's a cluster headache. Cluster headaches also tend to last under two hours and seem to occur as often as daily for several weeks, then go into remission for an extended period.

Paroxysmal headaches are also linked to REM sleep, but these last less than thirty minutes and affect only half the head. Women are more likely than men to suffer from these headaches. A woman may experience ten to fifteen headaches within twenty-four hours, each lasting from a few minutes to as long as twenty minutes.

People who wake up with headaches may have other underlying problems, such as high blood pressure, allergies, or sinus inflammation. Headaches can also result from hangovers or too-thick pillows. Someone with a bit of arthritis may extend the neck and shoulders even before bed and feel the effect the next morning. As someone who suffers from this problem, I can tell you there are specific positions that will trigger this type of pain. For me, falling asleep on the couch or on a plane or train brings on a headache the next morning.

Sleep Phase Problems

Most of us get sleepy in the evening at 10:00 P.M. and wake at 7:00 A.M., give or take a bit. However, for some, those hours of "normalcy" are a dream. Many teenagers and those in their early twenties will find exactly the opposite. They feel most alert around 8:00 P.M. and can't fall asleep till 3:00 or 4:00 A.M. Morning wake-up is awful, not comfortably occurring till noon or 1:00 P.M.! This change is called sleep phase delay syndrome. The opposite can also occur. Folks can't stay up later than 8:00 P.M., but watch out in the morning! They awaken at 4:00 A.M. This is called sleep phase advance syndrome and is much more common in the elderly.

However, there are ways to change these problems and reinforce a more normal sleep cycle. Bright light therapy is one (see box on page 161). Other behavioral tricks are to maintain a rigid wake schedule and force your sleep to fit. This can be difficult; light therapy makes it easier.

Sleep State Misperception

Some women may be sleeping quite well but *believe* they have a sleep problem. We call this sleep state misperception. People are convinced that their sleep is too short and of poor quality. They're often tired during the day and say their sleep problem is keeping them from functioning at their best. Yet when we do a sleep study their sleep archi-

Seeing the Light

Bright light therapy uses a specific form of light, emitted from a specially designed light box, which is as bright as the sun at dawn. Light therapy can be used for sleep phase delay syndrome, and for sleep problems caused by seasonal affective disorder (SAD) and by shift work. Before starting light therapy, you'll need a professional eye exam to make sure you don't have any retinal disease.

• Obtain a light box through a reputable firm. Light boxes are generally well-built for consistent light and proper reflection and shielding. You can rent these boxes through home health care companies or medical and surgical supply stores, or you can purchase one directly. (For some sources, see Appendix II.)

• The box should be 10,000 lux on a large field (12 to 16 inches by 22 to 36 inches). The larger and brighter the field, the less time is needed to obtain the light effect.

• Use the box for twenty minutes daily. For sleep phase delay syndrome, timing should be within fifteen minutes of a set, *consistent* wake time. For sleep phase advance syndrome, use the box around 4:00 or 5:00 in the afternoon.

• Sit within two or three feet of the light box. (Distance depends on the size of the box. The smaller the box, the closer you sit.)

• Face the box and focus your eyes on something nearby (the TV, reading material, a window) so that you're not looking directly at the box but light enters your eyes.

• You should see effects within one to two weeks, but consistent, daily use is required to maintain the effects. Only fifteen minutes of light exposure may be needed for maintenance.

tecture is found to be close to normal. They believe they awaken during the night, but in reality they don't.

For example, Anne came into my office quite upset because she had very fragmented sleep. She would sleep in two- and three-hour blocks between 10:00 P.M. and 8:00 A.M., sometimes awakening, other times believing she had awakened. Overall, she would obtain seven hours of sleep but felt that her sleep was very disrupted. She clearly felt that she had a problem since she was not getting eight hours of sleep.

When we spoke, it was obvious that Anne had locked on to this idea from childhood. Her parents had insisted that she sleep eight hours a night. Unfortunately, while well-meaning, this advice had the opposite effect because, biologically, she was geared to a six- or seven-hour night. As a child, Anne was put in her bed and told to fall asleep whether she was tired or not. She became stressed and anxious if she didn't sleep during the allotted time. So our task was to find the number of hours that worked well for her. As we talked and looked at her sleep logs, it was clear that seven hours of sleep was more than adequate for Anne. Therefore, she could sleep from midnight until 7:00 A.M. or from 11:00 P.M. until 6:00 A.M. There was no need for her to be in bed from 10:00 P.M. until 8:00 A.M.

If this sounds like you, it might be wise to keep a sleep log. Try to find your true hours of sleep. Try our simple sleep log on page 163.

Once you see the amount of sleep you're actually getting, you might find, as Anne did, that you're simply going to bed before you're tired. Or you might be trying to sleep too long when your natural rhythms are set for a shorter period of sleep.

When to See a Sleep Specialist

How do you know when you need specialized care for a sleep problem? Ask yourself these questions:

- Has your problem continued for longer than a month?
- Have your own trials of over-the-counter medications and other remedies gotten nowhere?
- Have you seen your primary care physician for a checkup, but he or she confirmed that there is "nothing" wrong?
- Are you confused about all this advice and at your wit's end?
- Have you had sudden attacks of sleepiness? (That's the most prominent symptom of narcolepsy.) Have you experienced sleep paralysis? Hallucinations?
- Do you snore at night and find yourself sleepy all day?

Your Sleep Log

Each line represents one twenty-four-hour period of your day/night schedule. The period starts at 6:00 P.M. at night and crosses to the next day at 6:00 P.M. During that time we are interested in the hours you sleep, including naps, when you awaken, whether you awake with an alarm clock or by yourself, and what activities you carry out during your wake time. These include meals, snacks, tobacco and alcohol, medications, and exercise.

That is a lot to mark down. Don't be compulsive about it. Just color in the box for the time you sleep. Mark an "A" for alarm; "M" for meals; "S" for snack; "P" for pills; "X" for exercise; "D" for alcoholic drink; "T" for tobacco. Here is an example of a sleep log:

DATE	6 P.M.	7 P.M.	8 P.M.	9 P.M.	10 P.M.	11 P.M.	MID-NIGHT	1 A.M.	2 A.M.	3 A.M.	4 A.M.	5 A.M.	6 A.M.	7 A.M.	8 A.M.	9 A.M.	10 A.M.	11 A.M.	NOON	1 P.M.	2 P.M.	3 P.M.	4 P.M.	5 P.M.
2/22		M	X			▓	▓	▓	▓	▓	▓	▓	▓	A	M		P		M			S		
2/23				D/MD			▓	▓	▓	▓	▓	▓	▓		M		P		M	M			S	
2/24	M					▓	▓	▓	▓	▓	▓	▓	▓	A	M		P		M					
2/25	M	M				▓	▓	▓	▓	▓	▓	▓		A	M		P		M		S			
2/26		M												▓		M	P		M	M		▓		
2/27		D/M																						
2/28																								

If you've answered yes to any of these questions, then you need to visit a sleep center. Ask your physician to refer you to a certified sleep center and give you a copy of all your medical records.

Begin to keep detailed records of your sleep problem (try using a sleep log), what happens and when. The more information you bring to the center, the easier the investigation. You will probably be asked important questions about your symptoms on the phone. That is why it is useful to call or be available at the time of that initial call. The center will probably send you lots of forms and questionnaires to complete regarding the wheres and whys of your symptoms. Here's where your own records come in handy.

Your initial appointment with a sleep professional will probably last one to two hours and involve a detailed interview to list all of your symptoms as well as your health history. It's important to share all the information you have, including any (and all) medications, even herbs, you've taken. It's also helpful to share all the things you tried but didn't find helpful.

What Is a Sleep Study?

If it is indicated, you'll be asked back for a sleep study. Some studies are done only at night, others during the night and day. What does a sleep study involve?

A sleep study is a way to examine various factors while you're sleeping. We expect that many things are different in sleep, and this is the best way of seeing those changes. The setup takes about forty-five minutes and involves the attachment of a lot of sensors to monitor you through the night. We attach sensors to your scalp, eye area, and chin to measure sleep. We also look at your breathing with a variety of bands around the belly and chest and a gadget on the finger or ear that measures oxygen. We monitor airflow through the nose and mouth with a variety of gadgets called thermistors or cannulas. Sensors will probably be added to your legs to monitor movement as well. All this is painless and boring. Many people fall asleep as we're doing it! All sensors are easily removed, and you can get up if you need to during the night.

After the sleep study, you will have another visit or phone conversation to discuss the results and suggested treatment options. Some centers like to see you and follow your progress. Others prefer to send information to your primary care physician and let him or her follow your progress, using the sleep center as consultants. A lot depends on your insurance (unfortunately).

Today there are dozens of sleep centers around the United States (see Appendix III) and many others abroad. You may find a good sleep therapist by asking friends or co-workers, by doing some reading, or by browsing the World Wide Web. Accreditation of the center or key practitioner by the American Academy of Sleep Medicine ensures standard care.

Research your symptoms on reputable Web sites on the Internet if you have access or by reading at your local library. There are many good books available (see Appendix I). You also need to become better educated about your particular problem and the solutions that may exist. The more education you have, the better health consumer you will be. And, in this case, the better you'll sleep at night!

5

In Your Dreams

Women's Wishes, Hopes, and Fears

A dream is a wish your heart makes. That's what the old song says, anyway. And it's not too far off.

There are two basic theories about why and how we dream. One is psychological, the other biological. But these theories are somewhat intertwined. Recent brain imaging studies have confirmed that the mind-brain relationship is strong in the land of dreams.

Let's take the biological theory of dreams first. For years biological researchers have argued that a dream is simply the result of random firings of cells triggered deep in the brain, which then trigger programmed firings along networks of cells that may hold memories. Depending on the area where neurons are activated, our dreams may involve an old memory trace or a new one, one image or another. Biologists would say dreams are all chance and meaningless, just our cortex or higher brain centers trying to make sense out of a lot of random activity.

By contrast, psychological theories have abounded for years. Sigmund Freud (the father of dream theory and psychoanalysis) and his followers long believed that dreams are ways to allow repressed emotions to emerge in the "safety" of sleep. Dream analysts argue that while we're sleeping the mind processes the day's events (or images from deep within our subconscious), and uses dreams to help us work out emotional problems, anger, anxieties, and fears.

Well, as I said, brain imaging work has reduced the need to argue about which theory is correct. Now there's a link between the biology and the psychology of dreaming.

We have known for some time that specific cell groups in the brain fire in REM sleep, and others are notably quiet. Imaging studies have confirmed this. Recent brain imaging work tends to confirm activation during REM of areas deep in the brain stem (which controls automatic and basic functions like breathing), as well as areas that control emotions (known as the limbic system) and forebrain areas, which coordinate sensory information, whereas brain areas associated with logical thoughts and planning are not activated. These are the higher brain centers involved in more thoughtful and abstract processes that occur while we're awake. So is it any wonder that our dreams are often chaotic and feel disjointed? In fact, dreams may be the point where the elusive mind merges with the physical matter of brain.

As we proceed, it is helpful to remember that just as women are different physically and emotionally from men, so are our dreams, reflecting more emotional intensity and less aggression than those of men. Since a woman's biology and psychology are intertwined, we may one day find out just *what* our dreams are made of.

What Dreams Are Made Of

The biological orchestration of REM activity and the dream emotions may be triggered very differently in the brain. Originally, dreams were thought to occur only in REM sleep, but we now know that dreams can occur in all stages of sleep, as well as in the intermediary stage of wakefulness as one drifts off to sleep. We know that one major difference between NREM and REM sleep is the amount of stimulation the brain can receive from the outside world. In REM sleep the brain is really separated from the outside world and from all sensory input, even temperature. In NREM sleep, particularly the lighter stages of sleep, we can still hear, feel, and even smell! Think of this example: An alarm clock's ringing can be incorporated into our dream before it actually hits our conscious reality and we realize we must wake up! Sensory impressions, including pain, thirst, hunger, even urinary urgency, may also help initiate a dream during NREM sleep.

We also know that much of the activity in the brain seen in an electroencephalogram during REM sleep is very similar to that seen when we're awake. We believe that activity comes from a very basic brain stem area (called the ascending reticular activating system). Also remember that in REM sleep we are essentially paralyzed. The only two muscle groups that work are our eye muscles and our diaphragms, which help us breathe. Our ability to move may well affect the way our brains weave a story from the stimulation they receive. For instance, how many times have you dreamt that you couldn't run or breathe in a dream? Dreams in which we want to get someplace but can't, or try to prevent a fall but can't, may be linked in some way to this very real paralysis.

We may have different types of dreams depending on the stage of sleep during which they arise. If you awaken people from REM sleep, most of the time they will report vivid dreams, compared with maybe 10 percent of the time in NREM sleep. Dreams in NREM sleep are reported to be shorter, perhaps more realistic and logical, not as vivid. But the data are conflicting. When scientists compare dreams of the same length, there appear to be few differences, except that REM dreams are more bizarre.

As I've discussed, some aspects of women's sleep are different from men's. Women hold on to their REM density—that is, the amount of phasic, rapid eye movements—longer than men. So you could say we may have more active dreaming. We also have more slow-wave sleep, stage 3 and 4 delta-wave sleep. Do we actually dream *more* than men? That's unclear. But we do have very different dreams.

What's in Our Dreams?

In order to dream, we have to have thinking processes, memories, emotions to draw on for content. Sleep scientists call these dream thoughts and pictures mentation. Women's dream mentation is different from men's. Our dreams reflect a stronger intensity of emotions and more cognitive activity. There's less bodily aggression in our dreams, compared with those of men. Unlike men, who dream most of women, we tend to have the same number of men and women characters in our dreams.

Almost fifty years ago researchers found that the content of women's dreams (as well as their ability to recall them) differed according to the phase of the menstrual cycle. For example, some women have more sexual feelings right after ovulation, so their dreams may be sexier then, too. By the same token, if you're more irritable and angry premenstrually, your dreams might reflect that.

As mentioned in Chapter 2, REM sleep is highest during the follicular phase of the menstrual cycle. During the luteal phase women seem to have more nighttime awakenings and more NREM sleep; they may also have less slow-wave sleep during the premenstrual period. Studies show that some women with premenstrual syndrome experience sleep disturbances because of upsetting dreams or nightmares.

Decades of research find that during pregnancy women report dream content that includes the expected child, and fears about labor and delivery. Pregnant women dream about their bodies and their changing shape, or animals growing. Their dreams are different from those of nonpregnant women, which seems to support the idea that dreams are related to situations and biological events in our lives. As I've mentioned, pregnant women also have more vivid dreams and more frequent nightmares.

Of course, it's hard to say whether a pregnant woman's sleep changes are affecting her dreams. We know that as sleep becomes more fragmented REM sleep or dream sleep may not be as condensed, so the sleeper may actually be experiencing some sleep deprivation or REM deprivation. Therefore, when the sleeper does dream, a very active rebound effect occurs.

There have been no specific studies of women's dreams in the years before and during menopause. But women do complain of difficulty falling asleep and frequent awakenings, usually caused by hot flashes. Estrogen replacement reduces hot flashes and increases the amount of REM sleep.

We see other differences in dream content related to personality rather than biology. The more intellectual among us have decreased physical activity and aggression in our dreams. But angry people generally have very aggressive dreams. There are also dream differences between patient groups, particularly psychiatric patients. People with schizophrenia and depression have fewer dreams, and their dreams are filled with self-negativity. Many people have recurring dreams or dream themes.

What's really intriguing is that dreams are fairly similar around the world. All people dream (even if they can't recall their dreams), and there are recurring themes (which I'll talk about later). Similarly, dream mentation (symbols, themes, and so on) has remained essentially the same over the last fifty years, in spite of all the major cultural shifts that have taken place.

Why Do We Dream, Anyway?

It was in 1899 that Sigmund Freud published *The Interpretation of Dreams*. But he wasn't the first to delve into dreams. Scientists and the clergy, among others, have been pondering the purpose of dreams and what they mean for centuries. In fact, debate is *still* ongoing over the origins and meaning of dreams.

Freud believed that dreams were our way of allowing ourselves to voice repressed emotions and unconscious thoughts. In dreams, he said, we could do things that we could not do in waking life and express strong emotions that we usually repress, such as lust, hatred, and jealousy. Freud felt that most dreams were linked to repressed sexual feelings. In fact, Freud used dreams to get at this repressed material to help his patients through psychoanalysis. To explore dreams in psychoanalysis, he used free association, a technique whereby the subject lies back on a couch and allows herself to think openly about any instance or aspect of the dream, to find out where it comes from and what in her life it may relate to. Freud, and others who followed him, believed that dreams are the best route to understanding the origins of one's psychic conflict.

While a number of Freud's dream theories have been disproven with our knowledge about the mechanics and the biology of sleep, recent neurological research seems to support many of his theories. As previously mentioned, brain imaging studies have revealed that areas in the brain linked to emotions and imagery are highly activated during REM sleep, while areas of higher thinking that we use when awake are not. That may be one reason why dreams during REM sleep are more vivid and emotionally charged than our NREM dreams or thoughts but not very logical. More important, recent research at the London School of Medicine found that patients who had lost function of the part of the brain believed to be linked to motivation and goal seeking also lost their ability to dream. So Freud may well have been correct in thinking that dreams involve wishes and desires.

Dr. Ernest Hartmann, director of the Sleep Disorders Center at Tufts University in Boston, is one of the dream researchers who suggest that dreams make connections and join areas in the cortex, the "thinking," problem-solving area of the brain that receives and passes information through networks of cells. While the basic structures of the brain are the same in all of us, each person's neural networks are different. So one person's dream will be different from another's. Dr. Hartmann also believes that these connections are guided by our emotions. For instance, we are happy, sad, scared, guilty in our dreams. Or we awaken from them feeling better or worse. In fact, he says, dreams may be contextualized emotion in which the most striking part of the dream provides a framework for a major emotional concern of the dreamer. This meshes nicely with the imaging work that shows activation of the emotional centers in the brain during dreaming.

Furthermore, Dr. Hartmann argues that dreams represent an explanatory metaphor, and their similarities of emotions or images, like strangling someone, or killing someone, may not be exactly what we want to do but instead be metaphors for our emotions. For instance, a common metaphor is dreaming of going through different rooms as we experience a search through our history. He also believes that dreams enhance old memories and weave in new experiences. By weaving together the old and the new, we can solve problems, relieve stress and trauma, spark scientific and artistic creations. Dr. Hartmann also believes that dreams provide a safe place for us to integrate a traumatic experience, make it less frightening and help us see things differently.

Dreams may also have a biological purpose. Some studies suggest they may help repair and organize the forebrain. Some scientists believe that dreaming is a necessary action in which the brain sorts and clears away unnecessary memories. We certainly know that the more college

Your Worst Nightmares

Nightmares are distinct from other dreams. They are defined as long, frightening dreams that rouse us from REM sleep. In some cases we might call them anxiety attacks that occur in sleep. And we remember them sometimes vividly. By contrast, night terrors are not technically dreams but are incomplete arousals from slow-wave, deep sleep. A person may not report a terrifying dream but may awaken in a panic, sometimes thrashing about, even screaming.

What happens during nightmares? The brain is very active, as in wake time. But muscle control is shut down (we are atonic). We're essentially paralyzed in dream sleep and cannot act out our dreams (although we may dream that we are running, flying, or falling). Our blood pressure and pulse surge, and we cannot control our temperature.

In some people the mechanisms of REM sleep can separate or disassociate. Aspects of REM can find their way into other types of consciousness. This is thought to be the basis of sleep paralysis and cataplexy. If the motor atonia of REM is lost, you may be able to get up and try to act out your dreams. This usually ends in bizarre movements and sometimes injury to yourself or your partner. You may have an argument in your dream and wind up yelling, or smacking furniture or your bed partner. You may dream that you hit someone in a dream and wake to find your partner has a black eye! (Did I say women have less aggressive dreams than men?) This is diagnosed as REM behavior disorder and is much more common in elderly men than women. But women can suffer the results of male partners' attacks during sleep.

Do you recall a famous painting, called *The Nightmare*, in which a devil is sitting on the chest of an unconscious sleeping woman? This is the sensation experienced by many people who believe they're having nightmares but are actually having what's called isolated sleep paralysis. This is another unusual event of misplaced REM sleep, but it occurs upon waking, or just before. The muscle atonia of REM remains and the patient awakens unable to move; her muscles still experience the paralysis of REM sleep, but her mind is awake. She hears and sees but cannot move. (She is not asleep and still dreaming, although it may feel like she is.) The episodes last usually only seconds to minutes, and the episodes can be quickly ended.

As I mentioned in Chapter 4, if you're aware that you have such episodes, ask your bed partner to touch you, rub your hand, or move your arm. Once your brain receives that tactile sensation, the episode will end. Or you can try to tell yourself to move your eyes or take deep breaths (which you can do in REM sleep). However, sleep paralysis can be a symptom of narcolepsy (see Chapter 4). So if you have repeated episodes and suffer from extreme daytime sleepiness, see a physician.

students study, the more they dream. So it may be that dreaming in some sense helps us process the day's activities.

New research at Harvard suggests that dreams may also serve a function in learning and memory processing. In one study subjects were trained and tested in visual discrimination tasks. Overnight improvement in the test was proportional to the amount of slow-wave sleep subjects had in the first part of the night and REM sleep in the last quarter. It may be that the process for memory consolidation requires slow-wave sleep followed by REM sleep.

Sleep may also help in learning by consolidating learning experiences. In another series of experiments, volunteers were trained in the computer game Tetris and sent home with tape recorders and sleep monitors. Seven out of the ten subjects who learned most quickly reported seeing shapes related to the game as they fell asleep.

How Can We Remember Our Dreams?

Wouldn't it be wonderful if we could make a movie of our dreams, then watch it at our leisure to explore its contents? Unfortunately, we can't. We can only try to remember what we've dreamt. And therein lies the problem.

Whatever reports we make of our dreams are made while we're awake. It's very difficult to know whether we've actually dreamt what we're recalling or whether we've woven it into a story while awake. We know that if we don't quickly attempt to remember a dream, it tends to be forgotten unless some piece of the dream triggers our memory. We must actually wake to remember the dream with full consciousness. Even so, we can seldom remember an entire dream (unless we've really trained ourselves to do so). Furthermore, it may be that what we remember and our interpretation of the dream memory is the most important part. So what you report of the dream may be more significant to you than the way the dream actually happened.

Typically, we don't recall our dreams because they're not rehearsed, they're not placed in our memory banks in a way that we can quickly recall them. But it is possible to train yourself to improve recall of your dreams. You'll need to keep a pencil and pad of paper by your bedside.

As soon as you awaken (and it should be a normal awakening, not being roused by the harsh ringing of an alarm clock), remain still with your eyes closed. Immediately think: What was I thinking? Try to recall or picture the thought that was just going on in your mind. Pick the most vivid scene in the picture and label it. Give it a title as you would a movie. That will help you recall it should you forget the starting point or climax of the dream.

Take the notepad and write down the dream as best you can remember it. Try doing this in dim light or with one of those lighted pens. Who were the main characters? What was going on? Where did the action occur? What place did it remind you of? If you think about it for a quiet period of time, more and more of the dream will come back to you.

To examine the dream further, think about what happened the day before. Many of our dreams build on recent issues and events. See if any of the previous day's events link to aspects of your dream. You may want to ask yourself: Why am I having this dream now?

If you like, you can buy a student's composition notebook and start to keep a dream diary to record your dreams on a regular basis. The more you recall and write down your dreams, the better you'll become at it. You can even practice writing down your dreams in the dark if you awaken in the middle of the night. You don't want to fully rouse yourself so you can't get back to sleep!

However, I write this chapter from the perspective of a sleep clinician who helps people overcome problems with *sleep*. If you'd like to find out more about dream interpretation, you can find two excellent books on women's dreams in Appendix I. If you want to do therapeutic "dream work" (as Freud called it), it's probably a good idea to work with a therapist or someone who is experienced in the field. Serious dream interpretation is not for amateurs.

What Can My Dreams Tell Me?

First off, since it's your dream, it's yours to interpret.

Freudian dream interpretation, or theories about the symbolism in dreams, even religious concepts, come from someone else. They can't take into account your emotions and experiences. When it comes down to it, only you can really make sense of your dream and figure out what it may mean in your life. A good therapist may guide you in that task but will not impose his or her own ideas on what a dream means. Similarly, dream symbols detailed in a book can only be guides for your own interpretation.

Everything in the dream is yours. Whatever happens (good or bad) in the dream is happening to you, or a part of you (or something you own or love). You should also remember that because dreams are your own emotions and your own stories, most researchers believe that everyone in your dreams could be you. So even though you see a dog, a man, or a child in your dream, it may very well be you or an aspect of you. A house in a dream can represent your body (or your symbolic self).

We are very self-centered in our dreams; for the most part we are everywhere and everyone in our dreams. For instance, I had a woman describe a dream to me in which she was watching her grandson and realized that he was her own son. Then she was holding a baby that was a combination of her son and grandson. Then she realized that it was really herself she was holding. Suddenly in her dream she became her mother. Imagery can be that complicated. So you may ask yourself: Where do I fit in this dream, and who are these people? Who do they remind me of in shape, sex, dress, feeling? Also ask: Could that be me?

Some themes that occur in dreams, such as flying or going to work naked, have to do with emotions, not necessarily with the specific situation. Flying is thought to be an act of freedom from the limitations of everyday life. Being naked (or in your nightgown or other state of undress) is usually interpreted as feeling vulnerable, exposed. See how "simple" this is?

Another thing a dream therapist will frequently tell you is that your dream mentation may appear to be the opposite of actual issues. So you *may* find opposites in dreams: good versus bad, safe versus unsafe. Rather than look so concretely, it's useful to turn the image around and see if its opposite is also useful.

Freud believed that dreams contain both memories of recent events and memories of things past in the dreamer's life, including events from early childhood that have left their mark, even though we have no conscious memory of them.

As women, do we dream especially "feminine" dreams?

As I mentioned, our dreams tend to have more emotional content than men's, less physical aggression (though sometimes we are the recipients of aggression in a dream). Dreams may be affected by how sexual we feel at a particular time of the month, how well we're sleeping, various stimuli in our environment, and even if we're pregnant. We dream about people who are important to us and may conjure up images of people we hardly know (like dreaming you are with a famous actor).

Many times women also will dream about their children and their life at home. Pregnant women frequently dream of the expected child or death or injury to the present child. This may be a way of resolving their excitement about a new child yet their sadness at disturbing the family placement of the present child. Often dreams will allow women to work out their concerns about the birth process or their commitment and ability to mother yet another child. No correlation has ever been found between the mother's dreaming and her ability to mother. I would think that examining her dreams during pregnancy would allow a mother the opportunity to explore areas in which she was ambivalent or concerned and perhaps resolve those conflicts before the birth of her child.

Women also tend to dream about social issues. In many cases, particularly in a work scenario where women are underrated or underpaid, equality may be a context of dreams, allowing women to sort out their feelings of inequity or support themselves and awaken with strength.

Using Your Dreams

• Keep a pen or pencil and a pad of paper or a student's composition book handy by your bedside. A voice-activated recorder is also useful.

• Get in the habit of thinking about your dream as you wake up.

• Give the dream a title as you would a movie.

• Ask yourself: What was going on in the dream? Who were the main characters? Where did the dream take place? Was there a theme to the dream?

• Try to recall and write down as many details as you can.

• When you go over the entries in your dream diary, ask yourself what recent events relate to the dream. What people? Why do you think you are having the dream at this time?

• If you have a particularly anxious, frightening, or angry dream, try to think of an event or an issue that may have sparked those feelings.

• If you have a recurrent unpleasant dream, before you go to sleep think about how you would change the dream. See if you can alter its content.

• To improve the quality of REM sleep, your major dreaming time, avoid alcohol before bedtime and don't let yourself become sleep-deprived.

Adapted from: *Crisis Dreaming,* by Rosalind Cartwright and Lynne Lamberg, HarperCollins, 1992.

There's also an interaction of REM cycles through the night, which may allow issues to resolve. This interaction can give us a clue to the mental state of the dreamer. For instance, over time a depressed person may change her dream mentation from gloomy to bright. This can occur even within one night and is frequently a clue as to how well the dreamer may do in recovering.

Dr. Rosalind Cartwright, director of the Sleep Disorder Service and Research Center at Rush–Presbyterian–St. Luke's Medical Center in Chicago, studied divorced and depressed people and found that their moods as displayed in their dreams changed during the night. Those whose moods changed from bad to better were more likely to do well without medications.

However, if you need antidepressants, be aware that medications can and do affect dream sleep. Antidepressants known as SSRIs, like fluoxetine (Prozac), sertraline (Zoloft), and paroxetine (Paxil), do not suppress REM but may dissociate some of its features, like rapid eye movement, and many people on these medications complain of increased or more vivid dreaming. Nefazodone (Serzone) actually preserves natural sleep. Tricyclic antidepressants do suppress REM, and they may produce a very bizarre first dream of the night. They can also create nightmares as a rebound effect once they're discontinued.

Sixty percent of people will have recurring dreams. Unfortunately, they are usually negative. I remember one patient, Cassie, who had developed insomnia. She was having difficulty settling down after the trauma of her divorce and noted that as a child she used to dream about rows of bathrooms. She would see toilets overflowing with paper and debris and not be able to find a clean one. This dream would follow her at different life stages, but it hadn't been around for years. She went into therapy and began to redream this ugly dream. Her therapist pointed out one interpretation: This was a very realistic dream and in fact it characterized her life at the time. Cassie was a person everyone dumped on and she had no place to do her own dumping. Fortunately, she used this dream as a springboard for changing her life.

All I Have to Do Is Dream

As Cassie's dream did, dreams can help us adjust to changes in our lives. They can help us accept health issues, body changes, or infirmities, learn that we are still whole even though our bodies may have let us down. People will tell you that after they've been injured and perhaps lost a function or part of their bodies, they still dream about themselves as whole, healthy people. Paraplegics dream in full body comfort and full body use. Many find those dreams are pleasant and fulfilling because in them they can act out many of the issues that they cannot address during their waking hours.

Can we brainstorm solutions to problems with dreams? We may in fact be able to make new connections that allow us to see solutions in dreams that we would not ordinarily see in the daytime, when our brains are overlaid with learned problem-solving techniques. So we have the potential to access other areas of our brains in a dream to solve problems.

Dreams have been well known to help people solve problems. For example, legend has it that Dr. Francis Crick (the codiscoverer of DNA) saw a double-helix shape in a dream during the time he was struggling to develop a model for DNA. Symphonies, images later put onto canvas, plots for novels, have all come to creative people during their dreams.

Dreams can also support us in mourning. Women may find themselves caught in that sandwich generation between aging parents and growing children. They will help a parent through health issues and then into death even as they must nurture their children. Dreams in such situations can help us sort out our feelings about the loss of a beloved member of the family—feelings that were, by necessity, buried during our busy waking hours.

I can relate to this personally. Over the course of my mother's prolonged illness and death, I was working, commuting, and caring for the emotional needs of other family members as well as supporting my mother. Her death occurred at a major holiday time and was swallowed up by relief that her suffering was over, sadness in everyone, and attempts to celebrate the holiday. I mourned, but there was little time for me to sit down and cry. For two weeks after my mother's death I dreamt of her nightly. I woke up exhausted, feeling worse than ever. Then the last dream came. In this dream I was working as a night-shift nurse at my training hospital. My mother came to me all shriveled, as she was at her death, with a child's red wagon. She brought the wagon to me and asked, "Can I stay with you?" I said, "Sure, that's no problem. Climb into the wagon." I wrapped her in her favorite blanket and pulled her through my workday. We went home together. I never had such dreams again. A friend of mine interpreted the dream to say that my mother wanted to be sure that she would always be with me in spirit before she left. I suspect I needed to know that, too. In a sense that dream was a closure activity that spanned two weeks.

In contrast, my coauthor tells me that when her father died a number of years ago she seldom had dreams about him, much as she wanted to see him again. But she says she understood. He was a man who did not dwell on things that he could not change and always advised his children to do the same. So she feels that he did not appear in her dreams during that period so that she would not dwell excessively on his death. Once her grief had subsided, he did appear in her dreams. It's interesting how we interpret these things, isn't it?

As I mentioned earlier, Dr. Rosalind Cartwright has studied the dreams of women going through divorce. She notes that those who dreamt about their spouses early on did better a year later than did others. Women who had dreams of anger at their husbands recovered more quickly than those who did not. Men's negative dreams tend to be about someone outside their immediate circle, whereas women's tend to be much more directed at their spouses. So perhaps these women were unconsciously using their dreams to work through their anger.

Can we make use of our dreams? Some people can. We call it lucid dreaming. In this technique, you study your dreams and try to direct their content toward a specific goal, such as getting rid of anger at an ex-spouse or being more assertive in your life.

For instance, therapists will teach people experiencing nightmares to battle back against the frightening figure in the dream. They may also bring this figure up in waking hours and do battle with it in an imaginary way or even a physical way so they can learn to conquer their fear.

Dr. Steven Laberge of the Lucidity Institute in Palo Alto, California, has done numerous studies on the ability to scan and alter a dream *while it is occurring.* He's been able to train people to recognize that a dream is beginning and to perform a simple task or change the phenomenon during the dream without waking up!

Dr. Cartwright has used a similar approach with depressed dreamers. For instance, someone who repeatedly dreams that she is being abandoned, or comes away from her dreams feeling defeated or depressed, can be taught to change her dreams so that she is in a more positive state in them. Dr. Cartwright has taught women who have been divorced or rejected by a lover to alter their dreams in a positive way. If the woman dreams that she sees her ex in a restaurant with a beautiful woman, she can alter the dream to have her partner see her in a restaurant with a handsome man. Such activity can free up negative feelings. It helps improve daytime thinking and self-esteem. You've heard of positive thinking. Why not try some positive dreaming?

6

Sleep and Sex
Where Do You Go After You Come?

Only in movies or romance novels do men and women have an endless night of passionate lovemaking and greet the dawn together.

You know the real-life scenario.

He seems to pass out cold while you're still hot.

But don't take it personally. This is just one of the factors that make men and women different *sexually.* In this chapter I'll try to help you understand what's going on. (For those whose partners are women, don't skip this chapter! It's important to appreciate how orgasms can interact with sleep.)

When Out of Sync Means No Sleep

Judy had been working with me for several weeks to correct some bad sleep habits that were leading to insomnia. She had been having difficulty falling asleep at the time her husband wanted to go to bed, usually an hour or so before she did (he had to get up for work earlier than she did). Through schedule therapy and relaxation therapy, she had been doing quite well. However, on this visit, she explained a new problem. "I now go to bed around 11:00 P.M. and generally fall asleep within fifteen minutes. Jim and I had enjoyed sex several times a week at bedtime. Sometimes it's just a brief episode because it's so late. I find that Jim falls right off to sleep, and I am left feeling absolutely wide awake, even if I felt sleepy before. So now I'm reluctant to have sex that late if it'll wake me up, and Jim just isn't arousable!"

This can be a common and frustrating problem for women. Here you are still feeling passionate, and the object of your desire is fast asleep. Guess what happens next. You're right, that initial loving energy turns to anxiety or anger, and the wake system gets fed! You're awake and annoyed.

I find that it helps to know we're a little out of sync with our male partners. We arouse more slowly and enjoy the heights of pleasure longer (more about that in a moment). That's the good news. The bad news is that when a brief encounter comes along, we may just be reaching our peak of excitability when it ends. Our slow cool-down period can be wonderful if we have attentive partners to cuddle and talk with. But watching our partners snore isn't always the most satisfying ending to even the most romantic of sexual encounters.

But let's not get angry. Rather, let's try other approaches.

Changing the way you think after lovemaking may help. There's something childlike about all of us when we're asleep. Look how vulnerable your partner seems. Look at what your lovemaking has done to him. Think of other wonderful loving moments, and slowly stretch and relax your muscles. That's right, start relaxation exercises and snuggle up. Before you know it, you'll be sleeping, too.

A change of mind-set not enough? Try scheduling a romantic rendezvous a bit earlier in the evening (providing you have the privacy and the kids are tucked in bed). This way you can both take your time. This may also help when differing work schedules make weeknight sex difficult. And "scheduling" can heighten anticipation and desire . . . always a good thing when it comes to sex.

The most important thing is to *talk* about it. Like all other matters sexual, many of us find that it's hard to communicate with our partners. Saying: "I wish that we could make love more often. But sometimes I'm just too tired. That doesn't mean I don't love you and want you. Let's find a way to maintain this very important part of our life together." Opening up communication between partners will help both of you rest easier.

Why Are We Awake?

There are a host of psychological reasons why women are wide awake after sex.

For one thing, women and men seem to approach matters of love and sex differently, no matter how long they've been together and how closely their personality styles mesh. Men and women have different styles of loving and being sexual, notes Dr. Bernie Zilbergeld in *The New Male Sexuality: The Truth About Men, Sex, and Pleasure* (Bantam, 1999). In general, men show love in shared activities (playing tennis, doing chores, and, yes, sex); women show love by shared intimacy (feelings), says Dr. Zilbergeld. That means words, affectionate behavior. So even though there may be physiological reasons why men roll over and fall asleep after making love, we may see it as turning their backs on *us*. We want to feel connected. We like men who are fully present and accounted for, says Dr. Zilbergeld. Women also feel more sexual when there's an ongoing romantic/erotic connection, whereas many men seem to compartmentalize sex.

A 1995 study of 541 male and female college students found that 36 percent of the women, compared with over 70 percent of the sexually active men, said they'd had sex at least once with a person with whom they felt no emotional attachment. A majority of the women said having sex made them feel emotionally vulnerable and able to bond more closely with the partner. This vulnerability may be another issue for us, one that promotes wakefulness. Can we truly be totally vulnerable, or do we feel we need to stay alert and "on top of things"—no pun intended? In contrast, a high percentage of the men said they had no trouble having sex with women they were not emotionally attached to.

So it's not surprising to learn that another recent survey of people aged eighteen to fifty-nine found that women were more likely to prefer activities associated with "romance," such as talking, holding hands, wearing sexy clothing, hugging, kissing and petting, and affection after intercourse. The men, by contrast, were more focused on the physical side of sex, trying new positions, engaging in oral sex, having both partners climax together, and looking at erotic movies and books. If the emotional connections are stronger for one partner, there's more to keep her awake, wanting to sustain the connection.

For both men and women, lovemaking involves a giving of oneself, relinquishing control and freedom. While it may be a romantic and erotic merger of bodies, sex is also a merger of egos. For women, this can open some very sensitive areas in a relationship, which fill our minds and leave us alert. You just had a disagreement, you've made up, you've made love. But there were things left unsaid. The closeness and after-glow of sexual intimacy seems like the perfect time to resolve them. But, again, the other half of the relationship isn't "present and accounted for." It's frustrating, and that interferes with sleep.

So now we get to the sleep issue. You've come. He's gone (figura-tively at least). He's sound asleep! How could he? It really has nothing to do with emotions. And men don't do this on purpose.

It's a well-documented phenomenon in many animal species. Stud-ies have shown a sleep-like brain-wave pattern in rats immediately after orgasm. It may have to do with the instant relaxation/resolution caused by a drop in the sympathetic nervous system's neurotransmitters. The chemical in question is norepinephrine, one of the stress hormones that promote alertness (the fight or flight response). This usually surges during intercourse and dips after a climax. It's possible that men have a bigger drop in norepinephrine than women, and so experience rebound sleepiness following a sexual climax. Women, as we know, tend to remain at a higher level of arousal after a climax, at least some of the time, and are able to have multiple orgasms. So it may be that our levels of norepinephrine are still high, promoting wakefulness. Or it could be the effect of intense body heating during sexual activity that causes men to fall asleep after climaxing. Even male rats do it!

Nice theories. However, the only study performed in humans shows no changes in sleep-wake patterns following climax in either males or females. Granted, in this study subjects were asked to sleep one night, masturbate without climax another night, and finally masturbate with climax. Subjects were told to perform these activities in random order, and still no changes were seen. Does that argue for interference from a partner? Perhaps. Or perhaps more body heat and energy are spent with a partner.

Sex: His 'n' Hers

Let's talk more about being out of sync sexually. The timing of men's and women's sexual arousal and release is different. A man can become aroused and climax in three or four minutes by physical stimulation alone. A woman's time from arousal to orgasm can be almost four times longer. Women generally need more stimulation than men to climax, including prolonged foreplay, kissing, caressing, and oral sex.

Women do have an advantage over men in that, once aroused, many can have multiple orgasms, whereas men have to wait to "recharge" after climaxing. This advantage may backfire, though, when we want to calm down and go to sleep. The stimulation for men dies down more quickly than for us. Many women also have higher cycles of heightened arousal linked to the hormonal changes of the menstrual cycle. Some women peak at midcycle or ovulation, others premenstrually (call it one of the few advantages of PMS).

We start to close this gap around menopause. With aging it takes men a bit longer to become aroused and sustain an erection. They need more foreplay and stimulation. Women, freed from fears of pregnancy, can be more spontaneous. So now we can both take our time and take advantage of the moment.

Don't think for a moment that older age has to mean no sex.

A recent survey by the American Association of Retired Persons (which now wants to be known simply as AARP) found that sexual pleasure continues to grow into old age. The first nationwide survey of sexual attitudes and practices among people forty-five and older found that although sexual frequency may drop as age increases, more than 70 percent of men and women with regular partners have sex at least once or twice a month. And two-thirds of those surveyed said they were satisfied with their relationships. There's more of a partner gap than a gender gap when it comes to sex in the second half of life. Women are more likely to be divorced or widowed; half of the women surveyed aged sixty to seventy-four lacked partners, and four out of five were alone after age seventy-five.

Women's sleep cycles may correspond to sexual cycles during the night, another link between sleep and sex. As I discussed in Chapter 1, during each period of REM sleep our erectile tissue (the penis, clitoris, and nasal membranes) is stimulated, and our dreams can be very sexual. It's during REM sleep that women may have nocturnal orgasms and men have nocturnal erections (and even ejaculation). If you think of REM sleep in that way, we then have four sexual cycles during the night.

It might be possible to take advantage of this cycle. The noted sex therapist Dr. Domeena Renshaw suggests a novel way to accommodate both your need for sex and your need for sleep in her book *Seven Weeks to Better Sex* (Random House/American Medical Association, 1995). She tells couples to pick a night, then set the alarm to ring an hour and a half after they go to bed. Get up, shower together, and make love. "The body's first sexual sleep cycle begins ninety minutes after you go to sleep, so your arousal level should be at its peak. The shower will refresh you, and the lovemaking will relax you so you can get back to sleep again," she writes. (She also suggests that if you fall asleep during love-making, don't fight the need for sleep. Nap for ninety minutes and try again.)

Trouble is, I don't know anyone who'd want to give this a try. Because continuity of sleep is important, I would not suggest fragmenting sleep further. So I can't endorse a middle-of-the-night tryst as a solution to your sex or sleep quandary.

But it may be very sensible to take advantage of that last REM cycle of the night, which usually occurs just before waking. Try initiating sexual encounters upon awakening, or after a good night's sleep. Set the alarm a bit earlier on a weekend, when you're more likely to feel rested. It's certainly worth a shot.

Not in the Mood?

It's easy to blame not being in the mood on being tired.

If you find your interest in sex flagging, there could be a number of causes (including low levels of estrogen and testosterone), as well as the effects of medications like some antidepressants or high blood pressure medications. If you find yourself unwilling or uninterested, blaming sleep problems could mask the real issue: poor communication with your partner.

Think about the situation honestly. If you have the sense that sex is the real issue, try to address it. If it's not, you need to address the issues that may be interfering with intimacy. In the meantime, keep sex out of the bedroom! There are plenty of other times and places to enjoy it. One problem in the bedroom is enough.

Some problems have to do not with sex or intimacy but with getting used to being a twosome.

Susan was newly married and came to see me worried about her husband's sleep. She wasn't used to sleeping with anyone and had been experiencing multiple awakenings. During one of these she noticed that her husband seemed to have an erection. She worried about this, thinking she had not satisfied him sexually. The insecurity was making it uncomfortable for her to sleep.

I assured Susan that what she observed was a natural phenomenon. Everyone, at all ages, has erectile tissue engorgement or swelling during REM sleep. It has no bearing on sexual need, although it may trigger a sexual dream in both males and females. Either sex may experience orgasm related to dreams. She had heard about "wet dreams" but didn't know what they were. They don't happen just to teenage boys.

Another sleep issue that affects couples is the fact of two different people trying to share the same bed. One partner likes the covers piled high, another prefers things cool. One person tosses and turns, the other tends to stay in one or two positions. In fact, a recent poll on "annoying partner sleep habits" by the National Sleep Foundation found that (next to snoring) the most common complaints were "wants bedroom too cold or hot," "hogs covers or pillows," and "takes up too much room in bed." Sound familiar?

In *The Clinical Handbook of Sleep Disorders* (Butterworth-Heinemann, 1996), the author notes that individuals who sleep on a hard bed tend to change position more often than those who sleep on a soft one. Young couples sharing a bed tend to sleep more deeply than older couples under the same conditions, says Dr. Antonio Culebras of the State University of New York College of Medicine. As age advances and the threshold for arousal from sleep is lowered, people become more sensitive to a bedmate's position changes. This results in more frequent arousals with smaller amounts of movement by a partner. His solution: separate beds might be advisable beyond middle age. If such a move benefits your sex life (and the quality of your sleep), I say, fine. Actually, I often find the most comfortable sleeping arrangement for two is separate beds pushed together. This way each partner has a bed (and blankets) suited to individual comfort while promoting intimacy. In some cases I have suggested totally separate beds (or even bedrooms) for some people with sleep problems (see page 192). But this arrangement needn't interfere with a satisfactory sex life either.

What Gets in Your Way?

If we think about it from a sleep researcher's point of view, romantic love could be just a confluence of intensely pleasant feelings that stimulate us into calmness and openness. And that aid sleep. What sex and sleep have in common is usually the bed, but that doesn't have to be so.

Anything that interferes with a romantic relationship can also interfere with sleep. Unresolved anger, stress, tension over finances, arguments about the kids. Your mother may have told you never to let the sun set on an argument. If you want a good night's sleep, it's a good piece of advice.

Not every woman wants to spend the entire night in a state of romantic rapture. At some point you really do have to sleep.

Both partners need to follow good sleep hygiene. A case in point was Angela. She had initially consulted me about her disrupted sleep. She noted that her sleep was most disrupted after romantic nights with her partner. They would spend a long time talking over wine and eventually begin to make love. She sometimes found it difficult to climax on those nights and noted that she would also awaken two to three hours into her sleep. She felt tired and grumpy in the mornings.

Angela was experiencing the results of too much alcohol before bed and, it turned out, before sex! I explained that alcohol is a depressant. It depresses not only wakefulness but also sexual sensations. Alcohol also changes the natural flow of sleep across the night. It prevents REM sleep from occurring until most of the alcohol is absorbed. At that point

Your Rx for Sleep and Sex

If you want a better love life, and a better night's sleep, avoid too much alcohol. As Angela found out, it not only interfered with her sexual responsiveness, but it was keeping her awake. Men also experience sexual difficulties if they overindulge. So think of a better bedtime luxury than champagne for two. I might suggest sorbet or ice cream, perhaps milk shakes for two (remember the sleep-inducing tryptophan in milk).

We've all seen those scenes in movies where people smoke after sex. Again, nicotine is a stimulant and will keep you awake. More important, smoking also causes lung disease, chronic bronchitis, and lung cancer (a recent study says older women are more likely to get lung cancer if they smoke). Not to mention an increased risk of heart attack and stroke. So lighting up after making love is not conducive to good health *or* a good night's sleep, and it will make your breath smell bad in the morning. And that's neither sexy nor romantic.

Angela would experience vivid dreams, as though her REM sleep was catching up.

This is called a REM rebound. Alcohol also increases the likelihood of twitching and body movements in sleep. These movements may awaken you for only seconds, but long enough to disturb the balance of your sleep. So many times people wake up in the morning feeling as though they've run around all night.

Angela stopped drinking wine late at night. She called to tell me things were much better. She even noted that her sexual difficulties were gone! Alcohol had made it difficult to reach orgasm. Even her husband felt an improvement. So we had killed two or three birds with one stone.

7

Sleeping Single in a Double Bed
When Your Partner Has Trouble Sleeping

When lyricists wrote about the music of the night, they most certainly were *not* talking about snoring.

During the twenty years that I have treated sleep disorders, I've seen hundreds of couples in my office. By the time they decide to visit me, things have usually gotten to such a state that the nonsnoring partner is concerned about only his or her *own* sleep, as in "Stop the @^$*&#% snoring so I can get some sleep!" or "I don't care if he or she has to sleep on the living room floor, I need *my* sleep!"

And snoring isn't the only problem that can rumple the double bed. Restless sleeping is a major problem. One study of sleep partners aged twenty-three to sixty-seven found that men tend to thrash about more during sleep than women (in one-third of cases, both partners toss and turn). Younger women complain of more disturbance with sleep partners, but couples, especially younger partners, tend to move more in sync (one rolls over, then the other). Not surprisingly, singles tend to be out of sync with bed partners. Sleep movements are decreased during a partner's absence, yet the partners say they sleep better with their partners.

Problems can also arise from differing sleep schedules. For example, one person's a "lark," the other's a "night owl," who crawls into bed at 2:00 A.M., or one partner must work the night shift and the other works days.

Sleep disorders such as restless legs syndrome, sleepwalking, and other parasomnias can disrupt a partner's sleep. But no sleep complaint fills my appointment calendar like snoring.

Honey, I Have Something to Tell You . . .

As many as 40 million Americans snore every night to a degree that affects their bedmates. In fact, a 1999 study by the Mayo Clinic found that people whose bed partners snore lose an hour of sleep every night! Women arouse almost twice as often when sleeping with a snoring bed partner! A study conducted a number of years ago in Ontario found that 86 percent of women said their husbands snored, and over half said that their sleep was disrupted by it, compared with 57 percent of men who reported that their wives snored, and only 15 percent said they were bothered by it.

In conversations with hundreds of women, both in and out of my office, the issue of "Just stop the snoring!" comes first. But how do you nicely tell your bed partner that he or she snores *and* that it disturbs your sleep?

Well, we can always try the loving, intelligent approach, as in "Sweetheart, I'm only worried about your health. Look what this magazine article says about the health problems related to snoring." A few snorers respond and find their way to my office. They admit that as far as *they* are concerned, there's nothing wrong, but if their bed partners are unhappy, they're willing to do anything to help. (Coincidentally, I noticed that many of these patients are in repeat marriages—seconds or thirds. Don't you wonder what happened in the *first*?)

In my experience, there are several stages in the bargaining process. The loving and intelligent approach fails. No matter how cleverly you phrase comments about snoring, your partner simply says it ain't so. The old tennis ball sewn into the T-shirt (see page 138) gets disposed of quickly. The gentle nudge (or not-so-gentle kick in the shins) doesn't seem to work for very long, either.

Next come anger and accusation—"You snored all night and I couldn't sleep"—countered by "Oh, you're such a light sleeper, anything could wake you." Then there's "You go to sleep first." So the non-snorer gets into bed earlier and tries to fall asleep while waiting for the

---

Stop the Snoring!

- Roll over (give a nudge to make your partner change positions)
- Use a "snore ball" (see page 138)
- Lose weight (even a few pounds can make a difference)
- Try Breathe Right strips or similar products to widen nostrils and aid breathing
- Try nasal sprays to reduce tissue congestion
- Use a humidifier to increase moisture in a heated room
- Avoid alcohol and sedating medications before bed
- Avoid sleep deprivation
- Try dental appliances
- See an ear, nose, and throat (ENT) specialist
- Consult a sleep specialist to find out if you have apnea (especially if you have excessive daytime sleepiness)

---

atom bomb to fall. Well, we know going to bed ahead of your schedule and trying to sleep doesn't work, so now we breed insomniacs, as in "You see, you can't even sleep when it's quiet!" We try earplugs, white noise machines, all to no avail.

Then comes the questioning: "If my own partner doesn't care enough to take care of his or her health, what does that say about our relationship?" Heaven knows where that smoldering thought ends. Somewhere in here, a separation occurs. Someone moves out of the bed! Ah, the question is, who?

Again, my experience has been that many more bed partners have been evicted than have been deserted. It must be far more lonely or uncomfortable to sleep on the couch, or in the attic or basement. The evictees may be more likely to come to a sleep clinic for help. I think it also tells something about who has the power in the relationship. It reminds me of the car ad where the couple argues over which radio station to listen to. The husband keeps punching up the soul, the wife a symphony. In the end the wife coos: "Honey, do you like sleeping on the couch?" And the husband puts on the classical music. Unfortunately, forced separation seems to be a common final pathway to help for snoring. But by the time a partner is spending nights on the couch, he (or she) is often experiencing other health issues related to the snoring or apnea, like hypertension and obesity.

Those of you who have success with the loving, intelligent approach, count your blessings. (If your partner is female, the chance of her snoring disrupting your sleep is probably a lot less!)

Recognizing Your Partner's Sleep Apnea

Snoring. Sometimes it sounds more like a freight train or the lion cage at the zoo. But more frightening than sound is the absence of noise as a partner gasps for breath.

Can you tell the difference between plain old snoring and sleep apnea? If your partner's snoring is soft and steady, it may just mean that there is some mild change in the airway. When the airway is completely blocked, the snoring stops and restarts with a loud snort or gasp as the pressure developed in the chest works to open the airway.

During the pause your partner may make a clicking sound as the airway attempts to open. Snoring, snorting, gasping, and clicking are all signs for concern, especially if a partner is developing excessive daytime sleepiness or suffering other health problems, such as hypertension. So make sure your partner sees a doctor, pronto.

When One Partner Can't Sleep

Partners who suffer with insomnia are another issue.

Remember the seesaw? If your partner develops difficulty falling or staying asleep, it's very reasonable to try to find out how you may be contributing to, or could correct, an imbalance of the balls. Stress, as we have seen, is a big issue. Is there a way you could ease your partner's stress? Is there a way to improve the bedroom setting? Subtle changes could help. A few minutes of mutual back rubs or a hot soak in the tub could do a lot to set a pleasant mood and reduce awareness of the day.

Help your partner review his or her schedule and improve it. Suggest activities that will take the focus off sleep. Take a weekend off; see if a new environment helps. Actually, I frequently recommend separate beds or rooms for chronic insomniacs as the best way to stop the cycle of poor sleep, worry, and blaming. I suggest they use a cocoon-like arrangement anywhere else, including the kitchen floor if necessary. Once your partner recaptures the ability to sleep, try a bedroom reunion and continue to reinforce healthy sleep patterns. I must tell you this advice is better accepted by women than by men. Women seem to like the idea of a "room of one's own." Men tend to see it as sexual rejection. Similarly, separate beds or rooms may open up a Pandora's box in a relationship. If it does, address these issues and keep sleep out of it!

If your partner's depression is the culprit, it is possible that insidious changes in circumstances (like job troubles) or your relationship have occurred that are beyond your ability to affect. Recognizing the changes and pointing them out in a nonaccusing way may be helpful. "Dear, you don't seem to be happy playing with the children/golfing/boating/ singing/et cetera, anymore. Is something wrong? Are you feeling okay? Maybe you should start with a checkup?" Help your partner see that a "healthy" report after a checkup only means he or she has to search harder for the answer. If symptoms continue, seek specialty care.

In the case of depression, sleep disturbances may be one of the few symptoms you may recognize. According to the Harvard psychotherapist Terrence Real, author of *I Don't Want to Talk About It: Overcoming the Secret Legacy of Male Depression* (Fireside Books, 1997), men often display depression in different ways than you and I, *if* they show it at all. Men are more apt to be angry, irritable (sometimes even abusive), or withdrawn (slumping silently in front of the TV); they may eat or drink too much; stay at work too late; have trouble sleeping or sleep too much. For men, Real says, there's a deep-seated shame about depression, which is seen as a weakness, as unmanly (big boys don't cry).

If you think your partner is depressed, your support for counseling and/or medication is vital. Don't diminish the chance for change and don't label your partner as weak. You may have to push your partner to get help. Keep in mind that it takes a very strong person to admit he or she needs help in anything (especially when it comes to men and their emotions).

What About TV Snoozers?

People who fall asleep on the train or bus or in front of the TV are sleep-deprived. Again, it's not a habit, it's an indication of a sleep problem. Either they're not allowing enough time to sleep, or the sleep they're getting isn't refreshing for a variety of reasons. And it can make for problems when one partner seems to be chronically sleepy.

Major life changes occur around a sleepy person. I say "around" because that person is frequently missing for decision making or important events. So, save your important decision making for when your partner is alert. Many sleepy people have bright times of the day—the early morning, after a nap, when medication is at its peak (or when it's low). Capitalize on those times. You may have to schedule events so that your partner doesn't nod off into the birthday cake or snooze at the theater. Short, preemptive naps may be sensible before important nighttime events.

Which brings me to another point. Yes, you can have different schedules for sleep. Some people love mornings; others love late-night TV. It's hard to mesh these two personality types and their biological clocks. One comes alive as the other one fades.

One thing you can do is make the most of weekend time. Spend the middle of the day doing shared chores and making shared decisions. That way you're at least on an even keel where awake time is concerned. Respect the need for the other to sleep and work to a different drummer. It adds variety to life, doesn't it? You'll take each other less for granted.

Safety First, Please!

I can't stress enough that sleepy people make dangerous drivers. Every year we read about a family wiped out in an accident on the way to or home from a vacation. It's usually a group with small children (who conveniently fall asleep during a nighttime drive), so Dad gets behind the wheel after working all day, falls asleep, and bang! Sleep sometimes happens when we least expect it. Let yours happen safely in bed.

Arrange early for alternative transportation home from a party, share driving; only do the driving yourself if you're more rested. That could

Your Couples Sleep Rx

Techniques to stabilize the sleep system (see pages 21–26) can be very effective in solving many sleep problems. However, one person's idea of sleep hygiene can be another person's hassle.

Face it, some people like to begin the night on the couch in front of the TV. You've probably felt that bringing your partner's attention to this habit will improve the situation. Problem is, this turns into nagging behavior. So ask yourself: Does your partner really need another mother? Isn't it reasonable to assume another adult knows what's good for him or her? If you don't need to discuss urgent matters at 10:00 P.M., back off. (Just remind your partner to try not to wake you when he or she finally comes to bed.) Make your partner's nap time your private time. Have a cup of herbal tea, read, call or E-mail friends, take that hot bath. Think of it as a respite after a busy day.

Don't get into bedtime hassles with the kids or your partner. Give others information ("Honey, if you're sleepy, why don't you go up to bed?" or "You know you'll be tired in school tomorrow if you watch Letterman"). Set the example ("I don't know about you, but I'm going to bed" or "I've got to get some sleep to be alert for my meeting tomorrow"), then see what they do. Okay, your partner may just say "good night." But why aggravate yourself before bedtime? Everyone will get the point when you awaken sharp and bubbly and well rested, and they're still groggy at breakfast. (However, teens' changing sleep patterns can be a separate problem; see page 212.) Teens' circadian rhythms are geared to staying up later. So maybe you just need to kiss them good night and head off to bed.

Relaxation exercises may help a partner who has trouble sleeping and, as I mentioned earlier, a soothing back massage can be very calming. A long, hot shower may do as well as a hot bath, and sleep-inducing snacks for two may be a nice remedy (see page 40).

A word of warning, however: Sedating medications or alcoholic drinks are *not* helpful for chronically sleepy people. They can dangerously worsen sleepiness. Alcohol and sedating medications prolong apnea and deprive the sufferer of oxygen. A shared nightcap will not help *either* of you sleep.

What about sex?

Well, your male partner may find sex just the thing to send him off for a good night's sleep, while you may be lying wide awake afterwards (see page 183). Then again, your partner (or you) may be too tired for sex (a common problem among new parents and two-career couples). Don't take either scenario personally. You have to *make* time for sex, even schedule it. It doesn't sound romantic, but it can give you something to look forward to. Try going to bed a bit earlier (or getting up earlier on weekends). If this isn't enough, it may be time to separate sleep from sex. I don't have to tell you that making accommodations is part of any successful relationship (and both of you do need to get the amount of sleep that's right for you).

allow your partner to take a brief nap. Travel in the morning after a good night's sleep, pull into a safe area and encourage a brief nap on a long trip, switch drivers often. Talk or otherwise safely engage the driver to help keep him or her alert.

Insist on taking over the driving even if your partner vehemently resists. Tough it out, even though your partner may be unhappy. Remember, too, that our propensity to sleep increases at the times our circadian rhythm dips, even if we're well rested. Driving anywhere between 2:00 and 4:00 A.M. is dangerous.

I would also suggest hired drivers for short trips, but please be sure you know *their* sleep schedules. Many times I find that "professional" livery drivers are operating on huge sleep debts. Riding in a limo belonging to another sleepy driver does no good.

When Your Partner Should Visit a Sleep Center

If your partner has had sleep problems for over a month and lifestyle changes haven't helped, seek specialized care. Again, symptoms of a sleep disorder don't tend to fluctuate. For bona fide sleep disorders, medical treatment may be the only solution.

The easiest place to begin is with your partner's own physician, not only because doctors know more about sleep than you do but also because they keep track of patients' medical histories and will be able to check their general health status (and your partner is most likely comfortable talking with his or her own doctor).

List the symptoms and the treatments that have failed. It's useful to bring an example of your schedules, but don't expect your physician to resolve that issue. If you've collected information on your problem, bring it with you, along with a list of symptoms. Some basic tests that may be ordered can include blood chemistries looking for problems like thyroid disease (hypothyroidism can cause sleep apnea) or iron deficiency anemia, which may lead to restless legs syndrome. Sometimes a viral check is indicated, since many postviral syndromes have excessive daytime sleepiness as a side effect. In that case, treating the sleepiness is in order until the symptom clears, usually after several months. For a female partner, a blood test to check hormone levels may be warranted (after all, menopausal symptoms can begin in your forties or even earlier).

If nothing stands out, or if attempts to solve the problems that do show up have failed to provide a better night's sleep, ask for a referral to a sleep center. This is not just a promo for my fellow sleep specialists. Truth is, many physicians haven't had much training in sleep problems. So you're more likely to find help for serious problems with someone who deals with them every day.

At a sleep center you and your partner can expect an initial appointment of at least one hour, sometimes with more than one professional. A detailed health, social, and sleep history is taken and physical tests are done as appropriate.

Following the visit, most centers have a multidisciplinary team that meets regularly to review the cases. Testing is decided on at that point.

The testing may include a night or a night and a day in the sleep labora-tory to monitor your partner's sleep. Once the testing is done, you should expect a summary of the findings. These can be reviewed by you and your partner in person, or sent to your doctor. Many centers follow you for many months, while others work with your primary-care physician.

It may be hard to convince your partner to visit a sleep center. The idea can be a bit intimidating, I know. ("You mean they're going to attach wires to my head and watch me sleep?") But some problems like apnea can be dangerous to your partner's health.

So keep arguing. This is one time it will be a win-win situation.

The Other Sleepers in the House
Kids Can Have Sleep Problems Too

Sleep problems seldom affect just one member of the family, especially when there are children involved.

Although many books have been written about getting your baby to sleep through the night or stopping bedtime power struggles with children, I thought it was important to discuss the sleep problems of children. The reason is obvious to any woman with a family: We are the most likely to be caring for a child during the night. And when the baby is howling instead of sleeping, or the three-year-old has night terrors, it's usually Mom who gets asked, "What do you think we should do?" or finds herself padding down the hallway.

Despite expectations that we should know or do those things simply because we're women, many of us don't have a clue about the nature of children's sleep and what to do when problems arise. Children can and do have sleep disorders. So you need to understand some basics about sleep during the younger years, whether you've got a new baby or a teenager.

What Do You Mean, "Sleeping Like a Baby"?

I can't tell you how many desperate calls I've gotten from mothers whose babies aren't sleeping well. One of the most striking came from the harried mother of a three-week-old. Now there's little you can do to help a three-week-old sleep better. It's unrealistic to expect structured sleep at this age. The new mom needs to know there's hope, but she must expect disruption for two to three months at least. That means, if Mom's the primary caregiver, she must be prepared to nap with the baby or run into dangerous sleep disruptions and sleep deprivation as well.

Of course, it's never too early to set the stage for good sleep habits. Simple things like light and noise can guide a child into appropriate hours of sleep. One of my first suggestions to sleep-deprived new parents is to read Dr. Richard Ferber's classic book *Solve Your Child's Sleep Problems* (Simon & Schuster, 1985).

This book has a wealth of information to help new parents learn the basics of good sleep and how to help their babies sleep through the night (so they can get a good night's sleep, too). Dr. Ferber advises parents to pick a schedule that's right for them and their babies, then stick to it. In some cases, he recommends letting the baby gradually cry it out for a few nights in order to eventually learn to soothe himself or herself to sleep without parental intervention. Not every parent can stand to hear the baby cry and not run to soothe him or her. But millions of parents say they've "Ferberized" their babies with great success. So these techniques are certainly worth investigating.

Although most of us are biologically equipped to develop good sleep, this takes some time. Babies are known to begin the rudiments of sleep in utero. When first born they sleep sixteen to seventeen hours over a twenty-four-hour period. Many sleep sessions are short, with the longest being three to four hours. Of that sleep time, 50 to 80 percent is REM sleep. So expect no more than three to four hours of steady sleep in a newborn.

By the age of four to six months, the baby begins to build adult features of NREM sleep. Slow-wave sleep becomes evident and eventually takes about one-third of a young child's sleep time. You should now try to regulate your baby's sleep patterns, with the most prolonged sleep periods at night.

By the time the child is twelve months old, she may sleep a total of fourteen hours a day. Most of this is at night, but there are two naps a day as well. The morning nap usually disappears between one and two years; the other may remain until age five. The quantity of REM sleep decreases a bit as the baby grows and reaches adult levels around age five. The quality of REM sleep, as we know it, does not begin to develop until age seven or eight, when the child is able to see and express dream "mentation" (thoughts and memories).

Although little research has been performed with young children, it seems that girls ages three to five have less stage 2 sleep than boys of that age, and perhaps this is the beginning of increased slow-wave sleep. The increase continues to be more significant in girls through adolescence. Whether this means girls' sleep patterns mature earlier than boys' is unclear since females tend to hold on to their slow-wave sleep longer as well.

So what's my advice for parents of infants? It's the same whether you have one or two (or more): Organize your baby's sleep.

I particularly remember a call from Bonnie, the rather frazzled mother of four-month-old twin boys. Twin A slept well; twin B, who had been sickly at birth and was still underweight, slept poorly and at a different time than twin A. Doctors had examined both boys, found them healthy, and implied that it was Bonnie's problem (a rather unfair thing to do). So Bonnie was understandably upset and not sleeping well, either.

It soon became clear that twin A did everything right (was a "good baby"), and so did Bonnie when handling him. Twin B, however, had Bonnie on the run. He cried and demanded attention. She couldn't stand his crying, thinking he was hungry or sick, so she constantly picked him up, tiptoed around him, and otherwise gave in to his every whimper. Consequently she was exhausted. Compared with his "good" brother, he was at least a "bad" sleeper.

Again, the first thing to do, whether you have twins like Bonnie or just a fussy newborn is to organize your baby's sleep.

Twin A's schedule was a guide to organizing sleep. (I stress the word *guide,* since each baby is an individual and may have different sleep development.) You need to establish a light-dark cycle (in this case, a shared light-dark cycle). At night it should be dark. A five-watt nightlight is enough to help you find your way to the crib, but the light should be turned away from the baby. Nighttime is the time for sleep or other necessary care such as feeding and diaper changing; there should be no stimulating play. During the daytime, babies need brightness as well as

---

Sleep Tips for Moms

- Make your *own* sleep a priority.
- Set (and keep) a regular wake time.
- Grab some strategic naps but keep them short.
- Get help with chores from your family; even toddlers can pitch in!
- Add some break time between the day's activities and your evening wind-down.
- Form a satisfying bedtime ritual with children, and for yourself.
- Check out that depressed mood with a therapist.
- Organize, organize, organize!

---

other stimulation: playtime, music, outdoors. At this age one can expect the baby to sleep in blocks of four to five hours with several shorter blocks as well. Mom and Dad's job is now to encourage the longest blocks at night. It is okay to wake a child in the day in an attempt to rotate the sleep times to night.

We separated Bonnie's boys until twin B was sleeping near the schedule of twin A. But soon they were able to sleep in the same room. Very important was that the father, the nanny, Grandma, and anyone else caring for the babies needed to adhere to the plan to remodel twin B's sleep patterns.

Since we are a daytime society, learning to sleep well at night and be alert in the day is important. This is the time to build sound habits that will follow the child through life.

However, most moms will tell you that getting the baby to sleep through the night doesn't ensure that either of you always will. Toddlers find their way into the parental bed, small children awaken from nightmares, and there's always the request for a 2:00 A.M. cup of water. Most of the time you'll all sleep soundly. But don't be surprised (or upset) at an occasional nocturnal upset, especially when daytime life gets hectic or unsettled. Prime times for these kinds of upsets are when Mom goes back to work or is otherwise less available during the day, or when the child starts school.

My four-year-old granddaughter (like her older brother at the same age) likes to go and "see Mommy" in the middle of the night. In her house that means looking at Mommy in bed, maybe saying hello, but not disturbing her, then sleeping on the floor by her side of the bed. The last time I visited and slept in Kersten's room, she crawled over me with her blanket and pillow at 3:00 A.M., said, "I'm going to see my mommy," and left. Even I wasn't an adequate substitute. Happily this behavior was limited to a few months; then all returned to normal.

Speaking of the parental bed, there are two schools of thought on letting a baby bunk with you. The federal Consumer Product Safety Commission in 1999 warned against letting a baby sleep in his or her parents' bed, citing an average sixty-four deaths a year among children under age two from accidental suffocation or strangling (including "rollover" mishaps). But sharing a bed is an integral part of child rearing in many cultures, and many parents feel it's a nurturing thing to do, even after breast feeding ends. Creative uses of bolsters or other barriers can help protect a young infant.

However, I do think that we have to teach our kids good sleep habits and how to soothe themselves to sleep alone. So use your good judgment, never let a child sleep in your bed if you are under the influence of alcohol or drugs or when you're extremely tired. If one partner is obese, please do use extreme caution.

So When Do We Do Bedtime?

A major issue with today's working couples is that their only free time with the children is in the evening hours (one of the reasons the concept of the family bed has become increasingly attractive).

Of course, evening playtime is stimulating for the child but necessary for family time. I'm often asked about whether late bed and wake times will harm children. The answer is no! Children need adequate sleep. When it is obtained is not an issue as long as parents understand that kids need routines and the grown-ups don't expect immediate changes. In other words, if you work and want to have your child on a late schedule of sleeping, the total number of hours is what's most important. Even if you feel your child is a short sleeper, you should provide encouragement and quiet surroundings for longer sleep periods. Studies have shown that those "short sleepers" really can sleep longer when the environment lets them!

Parents must understand, also, that when social needs such as school intervene, the child cannot switch sleep times without planning and time. Many families see this issue every summer. Children go to sleep later and later over the summer, then, suddenly, when school is upon them, they cannot fall asleep at regular times. This switch can only occur slowly.

Even with busy schedules, parents must help children make the transition from wake to sleep with soothing activities, like singing or reading aloud. The calming effect of these shared activities is often enough to help kids fall asleep more easily and stay asleep.

Television can be much too stimulating for young children to watch before bed. In fact, a recent study of almost five hundred children in southeastern New England found that the greatest sleep disturbances occurred in children who watched the most television each day and those who watched a lot of TV before bed (especially those with TV sets in their bedrooms). Watching TV seemed to delay sleep onset, shorten sleep duration, and lead to anxiety around sleep and bedtime resistance.

Bedtime refusal is a very common problem. This can take the form of bouts of crying, leaving the bedroom repeatedly, frequent requests for a drink of water, and so forth. Besides disrupting the child's sleep, such behavior can create chaos in the home. Some parents get so frustrated they'll let the child sleep with them, or even bunk with the child.

A novel solution to this problem is a "bedtime pass." This is the brainstorm of a psychologist from the famed Father Flanagan's Boys Home in Boys Town, Nebraska. Dr. Patrick C. Friman created passes out of five-by-seven-inch index cards and, in one experiment, gave the passes to two brothers, aged three and ten, who both had severe bedtime refusal problems. The boys were told that they could exchange the passes without penalty for one visit out of their room after bedtime each night. The visits were to be short and have a specific purpose, such as getting a drink of water, going to the bathroom, or getting a hug from their parents. After each visit, the kids had to surrender the passes to their parents until the following night. Dr. Friman found that this simple plan reduced crying and bedroom escapes from several times a night to zero times in both children! He's since helped a number of families adopt the bedtime pass plan with similar success.

Why does it work? Hard to say, comments Dr. Friman. He suspects the pass may act as a transitional object, similar to the security blanket or stuffed animal many children use to help themselves go from wake to sleep. (Studies show these "loveys" reduce nighttime arousals and help calm children.) Once the children had their passes, they knew that they could leave their beds and get their parents' attention without misbehavior, and perhaps that knowledge itself had a calming effect.

Bedtime struggles can become a habit, but so can sleep. To teach children "sleep alone" skills, parents need to withdraw. A bedtime pass can eliminate the struggles, the crying, and the guilt of "letting the child cry it out," and help kids learn to calm themselves in a way that's easy for all concerned. It's certainly worth a try!

Sleepwalking, Nightmares, and Night Terrors

As many of you know, children go through some "natural" phases that can create sleep problems. They are referred to as parasomnias because they happen around sleep, not necessarily *in* sleep. These include sleepwalking, and could also involve sleep talking, tooth grinding, night terrors, and nightmares. Such behaviors can be upsetting for *both* parent and child.

Sleepwalking is technically called somnambulism. It occurs following a brief arousal from slow-wave sleep, therefore usually in the first third of the night. A child with somnambulism may sit up, open her eyes, appear awake, then stumble around the room. The child may carry out a complex motor event, like opening a door or walking down the stairs, but there doesn't seem to be any forethought to it. There is seldom any recollection of these events, but injury can occur. Falls, for instance, on staircases (or even climbing out of a window) can produce severe injuries. I saw one child at my clinic who'd walked off the second-floor balcony of his summer home.

Although the motor activity is not planned, it can be habitual. So a child might get up, throw clothes around, go to the bathroom, or go out of a bedroom door as she would do in the morning in this very deep stage of sleep. Sleepwalking is much more typical with young children, and it tends to run in families. At least 15 percent of people have walked in their sleep during childhood.

The peak prevalence for sleepwalking is around ages four and five. We seldom see it after puberty. The causes are unknown, but we believe sleepwalking is just the result of neurological change needing time to catch up with general maturation. Should somnambulism start in adult-hood, we always look to psychological stresses as a cause and frequently recommend some form of psychotherapy.

There is treatment available in the form of drugs called benzodi-azepines (such as Valium or Klonopin), which lessen slow-wave sleep and reduce anxiety. This isn't always the first approach, however. If the child is in a known environment, sometimes only extra safety precau-tions such as locking a door or putting a gate across it, removing sharp things from the bed area, or padding side rails on youth beds are needed.

I have often recommended a rope with noisy cans on it tied across the room where the child may walk. The noise from hitting the cans may be enough to prompt full awakening in the child. That's the goal: safe waking and a return to bed. With older kids, I recommend an electric eye purchased from an electronics store placed in the child's usual path. Again, the noise of the alarm should complete awakening.

Night terrors are an all-too-frequent part of early childhood. The child awakens suddenly, usually within sixty to ninety minutes or so of sleep onset, and screams. She may get up from bed, run around wildly, enter your bed. She'll push off all attempts of help while screaming uncontrollably. The activity is generally very panicked. You are helpless to stop it and scared silly that something is terribly wrong. In the morn-ing your child has no idea what happened and why you are sleep-deprived from worry all night. Yep, sounds like a night terror!

This activity is usually the result of an incomplete arousal from slow-wave sleep into a "lighter" stage of sleep, or even a waking state, and is fairly normal at young ages. Young children have an abundance of slow-wave sleep and in some the arousal mechanism may be immature. As with most parasomnias, the typical age of occurrence for night terrors is four to six years old, but some children will continue until puberty. Most night terrors tend to run in families; the biological propensity to develop a parasomnia, to have an incomplete arousal, is strong.

The major clue that your child is having a night terror is that she has no memory of the event. If you find that this is true, do yourself and the child a favor. Don't speak about the activity in front of her. It can be very frightening to a young child to know that she's doing something she doesn't remember in the night and, worse, that it is scaring you! If the activity happens several times across the night or is more prevalent toward morning, mention it to your doctor. In rare cases these episodes are seizures. A sleep study can help tell the difference.

A major key to treating night terrors or other parasomnias is to prevent sleep deprivation. Sleep-deprived individuals tend to make up lost sleep in the form of slow-wave sleep, worsening the chances of having an event. Also, leaving a light on in the room or having soft music playing may lessen slow-wave sleep.

Dream Development

Many of us wonder what our children, especially young toddlers, are dreaming. The answer for the very young is that they probably are not "dreaming" in the way we do. In order to have a dream as we know it, a child must have the cognitive skills to construct symbolic forms of reality. It is fair to say, then, that little mentation is occurring until the child has conscious awareness about her own development and can separate herself as an individual from Mom.

Dream reports start around age three but are very brief, involve mostly animals, not humans, and have little movement, imagery, or self-portrayal. Around age seven to eight, children can really put themselves in a dream, if they have good visual and spatial ability. Now dreams are frequent, with complex stories, lots of movement, social interactions, affect, and self-representation. Therefore, we find that dreams are in a developmental mode and a formation mode through most of adolescence.

Why, then, do babies have REM sleep? This is an area of interest to sleep researchers. We believe that the neurological activity of REM sleep stimulates the brain cells in the visual or other sensory tracts for future use. This sleep stage may serve as an exerciser to lay down important neural networks. We also suspect that REM sleep provides a reinforcement for learning, incorporating lessons into neural tracts.

A word about nightmares: All children have them. Just as grown-ups do, children may use their dreams to work out problems. But bad dreams can reflect troubles in school or with peers, even abuse. So listen carefully when your kids tell you about their bad dreams.

Bed-wetting

Bed-wetting (enuresis) was once thought to be a parasomnia, a feature of incomplete arousal. However, we now know that bed-wetting can occur through various sleep stages.

Some children have a form of irritable bladder in which mild spasms trigger the bladder to empty. In the most benign cases, the child has an incomplete awakening and thinks she's in the bathroom, then urinates. If such episodes continue for long, talking with the child's physician is sensible.

Considering how often the child needs to urinate in the day and comparing the late-day fluid intake on dry and wet days will give you clues to preventing bed-wetting. Limiting evening intake of fluids will help. Many private companies will be happy to sell you magic solutions to bed-wetting. Essentially, they train you to anticipate the wetting or disrupt the child by alerting her to wake up before she typically wets. Eventually your child connects the signals of impending urination and, in theory, will awaken herself. This sounds good, but unless the child is ready, the disruption to everyone's sleep may work against you. Yes, helping your child recognize the feeling of a full bladder helps when she's ready. Eventually your child connects the signals of urination. Yes, offering rewards for dry nights can speed things up. But, in the end, her developmental schedule will prevail.

I hate to suggest that bed-wetting is a call for attention. But you know your child. Is she getting enough of your loving attention during the day? It's something to consider.

With a sudden onset of bed-wetting following otherwise dry periods, it's wise to check for other physical causes: medication changes, infections, and so on. I am a big proponent of keeping in touch with your health care provider. She should be a large part of your team approach to considering the right care for your child. For bed-wetting, imipramine (Tofranil), a tricyclic antidepressant, has been helpful. In low doses at bedtime this drug will increase muscle tone and may allow the child better bladder control.

Overall, if you can be assured there is no physical cause for your child's enuresis, it's best to say as little as possible and wait it out. Why add discomfort and negative attention to your child's life? Even small children can matter-of-factly take the sheets off a bed and place them near or in the washer. Replacing the sheet during the night may be possible for others. Eventually, the child outgrows the problem. Sometimes the less said, the better.

Sleep Disorders in Children

Can little kids have grown-up sleep disorders? Absolutely.

The most prevalent sleep disorder among kids is snoring and sleep-disturbed breathing. This is similar to, and in some cases identical to, the adult disorder of sleep apnea. Like adults, children snore when some area between the nose and lungs is compromised (or shut) cyclically during sleep. The most frequent cause in children is enlarged tonsils and/or adenoids. The tonsils or adenoids shrink the available airway and force the lungs to work harder to suck air in. Sometimes, the negative force necessary to get adequate air in collapses the entire airway. The child's brain recognizes that it's not getting enough air, and the child wakes up. Once awake, the child resumes normal breathing and goes back to sleep to begin the cycle anew.

During the process of opening the airway, the child grunts, gasps, or snores. Children naturally find the best position in which to sleep and breathe. Usually, while they are on their backs, their heads are thrown back and necks extended as a way to clear the airway: Many times children will choose to sleep on their hands and knees. This position may avoid some of the closures. It's estimated that 4 percent of all children may suffer from sleep apnea.

Tonsillectomy and adenoidectomy are frequently cures for sleep apnea in children. But make sure the surgery is followed up with a sleep study to confirm that the breathing disorder is fully corrected. The surgery may have cured the *symptom* of snoring but not treated the underlying problem. Read the section on treatments for adult sleep apnea in Chapter 4. A continuous positive airway pressure (CPAP) device can be used on children as young as four.

Unfortunately, even though most moms can give excellent descriptions of sleep apnea, some doctors think it will all clear up as the child grows. This may well be the case. However, your child may have significant symptoms in the meantime. Apnea can cause a severe loss of oxygen at night, a major insult to the rapidly growing brain. Kids with apnea may reflect the result of disrupted sleep by increased irritability during the day, which could be misdiagnosed as attention deficit–hyperactivity disorder (ADHD), mental retardation, or learning disabilities. Children who get restless when they try to fight their feelings of sleepiness could be labeled as lazy, troublemaking, and so on.

In fact, a recent study from the Children's National Medical Center indicates that children with ADHD experience a higher rate of severe sleep problems (and reported them once a week) than kids who don't have the disorder. Sleep problems included insomnia, feeling too keyed up to go to sleep, frequent waking during the night, bed-wetting, nightmares, teeth grinding, daytime tiredness, and falling asleep during the day. Not surprisingly, children with ADHD taking stimulant medication such as Ritalin had a rate of insomnia twice as high as kids not receiving treatment. Children on stimulants were also more likely to experience frequent awakenings, bed-wetting, and daytime sleepiness.

I have always been concerned that sleep disorders are being missed as a *cause* of hyperactivity. Hopefully, this study will prompt physicians to rule out sleep problems before a diagnosis of ADHD is made, and also cause them to think carefully before routinely prescribing stimulants.

Other sleep disorders can be seen in children of all ages. These include restless legs syndrome, or periodic leg movement during the night, and narcolepsy (see Chapter 4).

I have seen several children who had full symptoms of narcolepsy at

---

Sleep Tips for Teens

- Set a regular wake time, and keep it constant during the school week, within one to two hours on weekends and holidays.
- Your teen can't do it all on an empty sleep engine: allow at least eight hours a night for sleep during the week.
- Encourage your teen to eat sensibly and avoid dietary disrupters in the afternoon. That includes caffeinated sodas and chocolate.
- Ask your teen to consider an after-school nap (less than thirty minutes).
- Allow no TV, phones, or food in your teen's bedroom. No exceptions.

---

ages five to seven. They hallucinated and were initially misdiagnosed as schizophrenic. While stimulants may not be appropriate for every child with ADHD, they can make a big difference in children with narcolepsy. Unfortunately, some parents are reluctant to allow their children to take stimulant medications for fear of long-term problems. But these medications can make a wonderful difference when used appropriately, and helping a child stay alert to be able to learn is necessary for her future development and success.

I can only urge you to be an involved and observant parent. Seek the best for your child, and give her the best help you can. Most sleep disorders are easily corrected at this age. Your child deserves your help.

If your child is sleepy or acting out during the day, if reports of problems in school are frequent, if your child snores or gasps during sleep, ask for a referral to a sleep disorder center for a full evaluation.

Your Teenager's Endless Sleep

When adolescence hits, the same child who was up bright and early (maybe way too early!) for the Saturday-morning cartoons may not crawl out of bed until midafternoon.

Sleep needs among adolescents are poorly understood by the general public. Several reports have shown a high incidence of sleep complaints in the teenage years. Teens have difficulty falling asleep or getting up in the morning. They also experience vivid dreams.

Prepubertal sleepers are among the most efficient. Just about every moment in bed is spent asleep. But by the time the teen years approach, a child has reduced her sleep time to ten hours or less. Then, as adolescence begins, a biological shift occurs in the timing of sleep. Most teens are unable to fall asleep before 11:00 P.M. and won't really be out of their sleep mode until after 8:00 A.M.! This pattern appears to be worse in males. You can see how difficulties with school times and the ability to learn arise.

An international authority on sleep, Dr. Mary Carskadon, professor of psychiatry at Brown University, has demonstrated the change in circadian rhythm and the need for more sleep in teens. She notes that a teen's urge to sleep is greatest as her melatonin is about to turn off for the "night," and the drive to stay awake is highest about one hour before melatonin is secreted, just as with adults. So, in this seemingly strange reversal, if we considered only the circadian rhythm drive for sleep, the teen is most alert at bedtime and "dead to the world" at wake time! Unfortunately, it's also common during the teen years to see a delay in the time melatonin is secreted, so bedtimes and wake times are driven even later.

Remember, though, that there is also the homeostatic drive to sleep (see Chapter 1). This drive increases with one's time awake. So in the teen, the homeostatic drive to sleep overtakes the circadian drive to remain awake and sleep occurs. Eventually and usually quite late. Combine this with an early push to wake for class and we have sleep-deprived teens.

It is even more compelling to realize that the valuable hours of missed early-morning sleep may affect the teen's ability to learn. Work at the Laboratory of Neurophysiology of the Massachusetts Mental Health Center in Boston has shown that learning is affected by the lack of adequate sleep. The work suggests that people need both slow-wave sleep and REM sleep to consolidate learning experiences from the day before. The researchers hypothesize that during slow-wave sleep, information leaves the memory banks and enters the cortex, where a slow process of chemical connections is undertaken. During REM sleep the information is practiced and recapped, solidifing the memory traces.

In a teenager who falls asleep at 2 A.M. and must try to awaken by 6 A.M. for school, that last REM period may not occur and the prior day's work will not be adequately stored.

Additionally, Dr. Carskadon has shown that teens, even if they're well slept, will develop an adultlike circadian dip of alertness in the afternoon. It is unclear whether that reflects a maturing of the sleep system or actual loss of sleep. She has also found that even when sleep times were held constant through the prepubertal and adolescent years, adolescents were sleepier in daytime nap sessions. Furthermore, by the end of adolescence, teenagers might have lost up to 40 percent of their slow-wave sleep. Dr. Carskadon also noted that ninth- and tenth-graders who got fewer than seven hours of sleep per night had more depressed moods, lower grades, and more behavioral problems.

Today we're keenly aware that teenagers need more sleep than they get. When allowed to sleep as long as they want, teens will sleep in excess of ten hours or they'll attempt to make up sleep loss over the weekends (see the box on page 216).

Part of the problem is that because their sleep rhythms are changing, they don't know their sleep requirements. Another part of the problem is that teens are under a lot of social pressure to perform. Parents and teachers want the best for their children and often try to fill their available wake time with activities that will reinforce a bright future. This means extra courses, involvement in extracurricular activities, after-school jobs. All this is combined with teenagers' increasing self-awareness, natural sense of invincibility, need to establish their own identity, desire to develop a social life, and legal ability to drive.

For some this mixture of freedom and emotional demands spells disaster. The highest rate of motor vehicle accidents occurs in under-twenty-year-old males between the hours of 2:00 and 4:00 A.M. Remember, this is the time of our strongest propensity to sleep. When we combine this cycle with an increased biological need to sleep, social and behavioral issues demanding awake time, and inexperience behind the wheel, accidents are likely. Yet sleep issues are seldom addressed in driver education classes.

One of the public debates about sleep during the teen years involves changes in school hours. Most schools today start very early, thereby shrinking teens' already shortened hours of sleep to dangerous levels.

Early research on the subject suggests that grades improve when schools start later. Teachers will tell you that first and often second periods are tough because students don't pay attention. With a later start time, everyone benefits. Unfortunately, the economics of busing, school crowding, child care, and after-school activities are also tied in to this question. Still, we're seeing some positive changes among enlightened school districts.

If you would like to become involved in changing school times in your school district, look at models. The Center for Applied Research and Education Improvement (CAREI) at the University of Minnesota has carried out a number of studies and published the effects of such changes. They suggest that you not assume that you can't change school hours, but remember that the process is one of communication and learning. Changing school hours affects students, teachers, parents, and others. Everyone will have strong ideas on the subject.

Sleep Phase Delay Syndrome

The most frequent problem of teenage sleep is a shift in preferred sleep time. I am often called by concerned parents when their children are unable to get out of bed in the morning, get to school late, and appear sleepy through the morning.

My first question is: How does the child usually sleep at night? Invariably I'm told these teens also have trouble getting to sleep at a regular hour.

This phenomenon is called sleep phase delay syndrome. It's a shift in the biological clock, so that the teen prefers to sleep between 2:00 A.M. and, say, noon. There's nothing wrong with this schedule if it fits conveniently into the child's day. Unfortunately, in the early teenage years, this is seldom the case. When a young person enters college, how-

Your Sleep Rx for Teens

Ideally, teenagers need eight and a half to nine and a quarter hours of sleep each night. However, they seem to be affected more easily than adults by erratic sleep schedules and are more likely to stray from regular sleep patterns on weekends and holidays. So set a regular wake time and keep it constant.

The National Sleep Foundation suggests that teens not go to bed more than one hour later on weekends than they do during the week. Don't deviate from sleep schedules two or more nights in a row. On weekends, wake time should be no more than two hours later than on weekdays.

When your teen is preparing to go back to school after vacations, have her go to sleep and awaken about fifteen minutes earlier each day until she hits the desired sleep and wake times. Make these changes every day (even on weekends), and have your teen avoid napping during this process. While she's adapting to the normal school schedule, encourage your teen to avoid caffeine. Add good quality sleep to the list of reasons your teen should avoid smoking and drinking.

Have your teen avoid bright light in the late evening. In the morning, turn on bright lights or open shades or blinds as soon as possible after waking to help your teen reset her internal clock. Keep to the schedule every day (especially during the first few weeks of school). Practice the Four Rs of Sleep (see page 20). And urge your school board to set later class starting times for teens. They will see their students' attention and grades improve.

ever, she can often schedule classes around sleep timing, thereby extending the problem until nine-to-five work life begins. Many of us have experienced this syndrome; indeed, this trait tends to run in families. Hence we describe "night owls" versus "larks."

Treatment for this disorder is best performed with the teen's active consent. It requires setting patterns of wake and sleep, which must be consistently held. The situation can often be helped by bright light therapy (see page 161), using a special form of lighting that's as bright as the sun at dawn (10,000 Lux). The child sits three feet in front of a set of lights for twenty minutes very soon after waking. The regimen is: (1) wake up at a set time seven days a week; (2) sit focusing toward the light for twenty minutes; (3) keep a regular sleep schedule; (4) avoid naps.

Change with this system is very rapid, but unfortunately it needs consistent schedules to remain in effect. Even one night off will disrupt the process. Therefore, the teenager has to be motivated to change.

Parasomnias in Teenagers

Parasomnias in teens are much the same as in younger children. However, in this age group it may be more sensible to treat problems pharmacologically. Many teens avoid activities like summer camp or sleeping over at a friend's for fear of sleepwalking or bed-wetting. For those nights, medication may be the answer. The teen can use the medication for a few nights or even weeks and feel relaxed. Education for your teen may also be helpful. It's important to know that research has shown a correlation between the amount of caffeine consumed and the prevalence of parasomnias like sleepwalking and teeth grinding. Limiting the amount of caffeine may work magic. Caffeine can be found in a number of foods and beverages other than coffee (see pages 33–34), including sodas and chocolate, staples of the teen years. If your teen becomes aware that these foods may cause a potentially embarrassing problem, she's more likely to avoid them than if you nag. You might want to switch to decaf coffee and noncaffeinated beverages yourself.

If your teen continues to suffer from nightmares or night terrors, it may be worth a consultation with a child psychiatrist or other mental health specialist to identify fears, depression, or stressors you might be unaware of.

With teenagers (as with partners), it's important to remember that everyone sets her own pace. Nagging about bedtimes only creates friction. Just as with any issue during these years, pick your battles wisely. Figure out what's truly important to you. Are you more concerned about weekday bedtimes or weekend curfews, for example? The more you can cut down on tension and stress during these years, the better *you'll* sleep.

Afterword

We hope you have enjoyed reading this book as much as we enjoyed writing it. We learned a lot in the process, too. You now have a taste of what sleep can offer you, and what sleep is all about. Trust us, it is only the barest of tastes.

If you want to learn more, the appendixes that follow are for you. We've included a bibliography of the scientific papers we discussed. We've also listed other reading materials, Web sites, and support groups that offer additional information.

For those of you who have spotted a problem, Appendix III lists sleep centers across the United States. This list includes the centers certified by the American Academy of Sleep Medicine. Many other centers exist, some very good and some not so good. To be sure of their quality, make certain that at least the center director is certified by the academy.

We wish you pleasant dreams.

Appendix I

ADDITIONAL READING

Sleep Medicine

Sonia Ancoli-Israel, *All I Want Is a Good Night's Sleep.* Mosby, 1996.

George J. Cohen, ed., *The American Academy of Pediatrics Guide to Your Child's Sleep.* Villard, 1999.

William C. Dement and Christopher Vaughan, *The Promise of Sleep.* Delacorte Press, 1999.

Richard C. Ferber, *Solve Your Child's Sleep Problems.* Simon & Schuster, 1985.

Peter Hauri and Shirley Linde, *No More Sleepless Nights.* John Wiley, 1996.

Lynne Lamberg, *Bodyrhythms: Chronobiology and Peak Performance.* William Morrow & Company, 1994.

James Maas, *Power Sleep: How to Prepare Your Mind for Peak Performance.* Villard, 1998.

Jodi A. Mindell, *Sleeping Through the Night: How Infants, Toddlers, and Their Parents Can Get a Good Night's Sleep.* HarperCollins, 1997.

Elizabeth A. Mitler and Merrill M. Mitler, *101 Questions About Sleep and Dreams.* Sleep and Wake Foundation, 1999.

Anne Remmes and Roxanne Nelson, *If You Think You Have a Sleep Disorder.* Dell Mental Health Guides, 1998.

Michael Smolensky, Ph.D. and Lynne Lamberg, *The Body Clock Guide to Health: How to Use Your Body's Natural Clock to Fight Illness and Achieve Maximum Health.* Henry Holt, 2000.

Gary K. Zammit, *Good Nights: How to Stop Sleep Deprivation, Overcome Insomnia, and Get the Sleep You Need.* Andrews McMeel, 1998.

Dreams

Rosalind Cartwright and Lynne Lamberg, *Crisis Dreaming.* HarperCollins, 1992.

Sigmund Freud, *The Interpretation of Dreams.* Reprint; 1999.

Lucy Goodson, *The Dreams of Women: Exploring and Interpreting Women's Dreams.* Reprint; Berkley, 1997.

Karen A. Signell and Riane Eisler, *Wisdom of the Heart: Working with Women's Dreams.* Fromm International, 1998.

Pregnancy/Infertility

The Mayo Clinic Complete Book of Pregnancy, Childbirth, and Baby's First Year. William Morrow, 1995.

The Staff of RESOLVE, with Diane Aronson, Executive Director, *Resolving Infertility: Understanding the Options and Choosing Solutions When You Want to Have a Baby.* HarperCollins, 1999.

Perimenopause and Menopause

James E. Huston and Darlene Lanka, *Perimenopause: Changes in Women's Health After Thirty-five.* New Harbinger, 1997.

Mary Jane Minkin and Carol V. Wright, *What Every Woman Needs to Know About Menopause: The Years Before, During, and After.* Yale University Press, 1996.

Geoffrey Redmond, *The Good News About Women's Hormones: Complete Information and Proven Solutions for the Most Common Hormonal Problems.* Warner Books, 1995.

Judith Reichman, *I'm Too Young to Get Old.* Times Books, 1998.

Nina Shandler, *Estrogen: The Natural Way.* Villard, 1997.

Bladder Problems

Cheryle B. Gartley, ed., *Managing Incontinence: A Guide to Living with Loss of Bladder Control.* Jameson Books, 1985.

Diane Kaschack Newman, Mary K. Dzurinko, and Ananias C. Dionko, *The Urinary Incontinence Sourcebook.* Lowell House, 1999.

Kristene E. Whitmore, *Overcoming Bladder Disorders.* HarperCollins, 1990.

Women's Mental Health

Rita Baron-Faust, *Mental Wellness for Women.* William Morrow/Quill, 1998.

Karen R. Kleinman and Valerie D. Raskin, *This Isn't What I Expected: Overcoming Post-Partum Depression.* Bantam, 1995.

Valerie Davis Raskin, *When Words Are Not Enough: The Women's Prescription for Depression and Anxiety.* Broadway Books, 1997.

Headaches

Alexander Mauskop and Marietta Abrams Brill, *The Headache Alternative: A Neurologist's Guide to Drug-Free Relief.* Dell, 1997.

Alan M. Rapoport and Fred D. Sheftell, *Headache Relief for Women: How You Can Manage and Prevent Pain.* Little, Brown, 1995.

Arthritis, Autoimmune Diseases, and Pain Syndromes

Leonid Gordin and Craig Weatherby, *The Arthritis Bible: A Comprehensive Guide to Alternative Therapies and Conventional Treatments for Arthritic Diseases Including Osteoarthritis, Rheumatoid Arthritis, Gout, Fibromyalgia, and More.* Inner Traditions, 1999.

Robert G. Lahita and Robert H. Phillips, *Lupus: Everything You Need to Know.* Avery, 1999.

Harris H. McIlwain and Debra Fulghum Bruce, *The Fibromyalgia Handbook.* Owl, 1996.

Paul O'Connor, *Multiple Sclerosis: The Facts You Need.* Firefly, 1999.

Devin J. Starlanyl and Mary Ellen Copeland, *Fibromyalgia and Chronic Myofascial Pain Syndrome: A Survival Manual.* New Harbinger, 1996.

Daniel J. Wallace, *Lupus Book: A Guide for Patients and Their Families,* rev. ed. Oxford University Press, 1999.

Sexuality

Barbara Keesling, *Discover Your Sensual Potential: A Woman's Guide to Guaranteed Satisfaction.* HarperCollins, 1999.

Domeena Renshaw, *Seven Weeks to Better Sex.* Random House/American Medical Association, 1995.

Bernie Zilbergeld, *The New Male Sexuality: The Truth About Men, Sex, and Pleasure.* Bantam, 1999.

Appendix II

RESOURCES, SUPPORT GROUPS, AND WEB PAGES

Many things can affect a woman's sleep, from hormonal factors like pregnancy and menopause to depression, pain, and chronic disease, including arthritis and cancer. What follows is a listing of resources and self-help groups that can help a woman cope with sleep problems, whether it's a sleep disorder or headaches.

SLEEP MEDICINE

Sleep Medicine Home Page
c/o Michael Thorpy, M.D.
Montefiore Medical Center, NY
www.users.cloud9net/~Thorpy/

The Sleep Well
www.stanford.edu/~dement/

National Organization for Rare Disorders (NORD)
www.nord-rdb.org

National Sleep Foundation (NSF)
1522 K St., N.W. #510
Washington, DC 20005
(202) 341-3471 fax: (202) 341-3472
www.sleepfoundation.org

American Academy of Sleep Medicine (AASM)
6301 Bandel Rd. Suite 101
Rochester, MN 55901
(507) 287-6006 fax: (507) 287-6008
www.aasmnet.org

Sleep Research Society (SRS)
6301 Bandel Rd. Suite 101
Rochester, MN 55901
(507) 285-4384 fax: (507) 287-6008
www.sro.org

World Federation for Sleep Research Societies
c/o Michael Chase, Ph.D.
Brain Research Institute
UCLA School of Medicine

Center for the Health Sciences
43-367
Los Angeles, CA 90095-1746
(310) 825-3417 fax: (310) 206-3499
www.wfsrs.org

NARCOLEPSY

Narcolepsy Network Inc.
(national office)
Reed Hartman Corporate Center
10921 Reed Hartman Highway
Cincinnati, OH 45242
(513) 891-3522 fax: (513) 891-3836
E-mail: narnet@aol.com
www.narcolepsynetwork.org

National Narcolepsy Registry
NSF and Montefiore Medical Center
(202) 347-3471

Center for Narcolepsy
Stanford University
(650) 725-6512
www.med.stanford.edu/school/
    psychiatry/narcolepsy/index

RESTLESS LEGS SYNDROME

**Restless Legs Syndrome Foundation,
    Inc.**
819 Second St. S.W.
Rochester, MN 55902
www.RLS.org

SLEEP APNEA

American Sleep Apnea Association
A.W.A.K.E. Network
1424 K Street, N.W., Suite 302
Washington, DC 20005

(202) 293-3650 fax: (202) 293-3656
E-mail: asaa@sleepapnea.org
www.sleepapnea.org

AUTOIMMUNE DISEASES

**American Autoimmune Related
    Diseases Association, Inc.**
Michigan National Building
22100 Gratiot Avenue
East Detroit, MI 48021
(800) 598-4668
www.aarda.org

ARTHRITIS

Arthritis Foundation
1330 West Peachtree St.
Atlanta, GA 30309
(404) 872-7100
(800) 933-0032

**National Institutes of Arthritis,
    Musculoskeletal and Skin
    Diseases**

National Institutes of Health
Building 31, Room 4C05
Bethesda, MD 20892
(301) 496-8188

American College of Rheumatology
60 Executive Park South, Suite 150
Atlanta, GA 30329
(800) 346-4753

CANCER

American Cancer Society
(national office)
1599 Clifton Road, N.E.
Atlanta, GA 30329

(404) 320-3333
www.cancer.org
ACS toll-free hotline
(1-800-ACS-2345)

**National Cancer Institute
  Information Service
National Institutes of Health**
Bethesda, MD 20205
(1-800-4-CANCER)
Alaska: 1-800-638-6070
Hawaii: (808) 524-1234

**National Coalition for Cancer
  Survivorship**
1010 Wayne Avenue, 5th floor,
Silver Spring, MD 20910
(301) 650-8868

Cancer Care, Inc.
(national office)
1180 Avenue of the Americas
New York, NY 10036
(212) 221-3300
http://cancercareinc.org
Counseling Line
(800) 813-HOPE (4673)

CHRONIC FATIGUE SYNDROME

CFIDS Association
P.O. Box 220398
Charlotte, NC 28222
(800) 442-3437
www.cfids.org

DOMESTIC VIOLENCE/POST TRAUMATIC STRESS

National Domestic Violence Hotline
(800) 799-SAFE (7233)
(800) 787-3224 (TDD)

**National Organization for Victim
  Assistance (NOVA)**
1757 Park Road, N.W.
Washington, DC 20010
(800) TRY-NOVA

**Eye Movement Desensitization and
  Reprocessing (EMDR)**
P.O. Box 51010
Pacific Grove, CA 93950
(408) 372-3900 fax: (408) 647-9881
www.emdr.com

FIBROMYALGIA

**American Fibromyalgia Syndrome
  Association, Inc.**
6380 East Tanque Verde, Suite D
Tucson, AZ 85715
(520) 733-1570
www.AFSAfund.org

INCONTINENCE/OVERACTIVE BLADDER

National Enuresis Society
777 Forest La., Suite C-737
Dallas, TX
1-800-NES-8080
www.peds.umn.edu/centers/NES/

**The Simon Foundation for
  Continence**
P.O. Box 815
Wilmette, IL 60091
(800) 237-4666

**National Association for Continence
  (NAFC)**
P.O. Box 8310
Spartanburg, SC 29305
(800) BLADDER (252-3337)
http://www.nafc.org/

American Foundation for Urologic Disease
300 West Pratt Street, Suite 401
Baltimore, MD 21201
(800) 242-2383
(410) 727-2908

American Urogynecologic Society
401 North Michigan Avenue
Chicago, IL 60611-4267
(312) 644-6610

International Foundation for Bowel Dysfunction (IFBD)
P.O. Box 17864
Milwaukee, WI 53217
(414) 241-9479

National Kidney and Urologic Diseases Information Clearinghouse
3 Information Way
Bethesda, MD 20892
(301) 654-4415
http://www.niddk.nih.gov/

LIGHT THERAPY

Society for Light Treatment and Biological Rhythms
842 Howard Avenue
New Haven, CT 06519
Fax: (203) 764-4324
http://www.sltbr.org

MENOPAUSE AND BEYOND

North American Menopause Society
c/o University Hospitals of Cleveland
Department of OB/GYN
11100 Euclid Avenue

Cleveland, OH
(216) 844-8748 (provides names of local specialists)
http://www.menopause.com

American Association of Retired Persons (AARP)
1909 K Street, N.W.
Washington, DC 20024
(202) 872-4700
http://www.aarp.org/

American Society on Aging
833 Market Street, Suite 511
San Francisco, CA 94103
(800) 537-9728

MENTAL HEALTH ISSUES

National Institute of Mental Health (NIMH)
Information Resources and Inquiries Branch
5600 Fishers Lane, Room 15-C-105
Rockville, MD 20807
(301) 443-4515
http://gopher.nimh.nih.gov

National Mental Health Association (NMHA)
1021 Prince Street
Alexandria, VA 22314-2971
(800) 969-NMHA
http://www.worldcorp.com.dc-online/nmha

National Alliance for the Mentally Ill (NAMI)
2101 Wilson Boulevard, Suite 302
Arlington, VA 22201
(703) 524-7600
http://www.cais.net/vikings/nami

The Anxiety Disorders Association of America
6000 Executive Boulevard, Suite 513
Rockville, MD 20852
(301) 231-5484
http:/www.users.interport.net/~lindy/adaa.html

Depression Awareness, Recognition, Treatment (D/ART) Program
National Institute of Mental Health
5600 Fishers Lane
Rockville, MD 20807
(800) 421-4211

MULTIPLE SCLEROSIS

National Multiple Sclerosis Society
205 East 42nd Street
New York, NY 10017
(212) 986-3240

POST-PARTUM DEPRESSION

Depression After Delivery
P.O. Box 1282
Morrisville, PA 19067
(800) 944-4PPD

Post-Partum Support International
927 North Kellogg Avenue
Santa Barbara, CA 93111
(805) 967-7636

SEXUALITY

American Association of Sex Educators, Counselors and Therapists
435 N. Michigan Avenue, Suite 1717
Chicago, IL 60611-4067

Sex Information and Education Council of the U.S.
130 West 42nd Street, Suite 350
New York, NY 10036
(212) 817-9770
http://www.siecus.org/

SYSTEMIC LUPUS ERYTHEMATOSIS (SLE)

Lupus Foundation of America
1300 Piccard Dr., Suite 200
Rockville, MD 20850
(800) 558-0121
(301) 670-9292
http://www.lupus.org/

S.L.E. Foundation
(a chapter of the Lupus Foundation of America)
149 Madison Avenue, Suite 608
New York, NY 10016
(212) 685-4118

WOMEN'S HEALTH

Society for the Advancement of Women's Health Research
1920 L Street, N.W., Suite 510
Washington, DC 20036
(202) 223-8224
http://www.womens-health.org

Women's Health Initiative
U.S. Department of Health and Human Services
Public Health Services, National Institutes of Health
Federal Building, Room 6A09
Bethesda, MD 20892
(800) 549-6636

National Women's Health Resource Center
2440 M Street, N.W., Suite 325
Washington, DC 20037
(202) 293-6045 (9:00 A.M.–3:00 P.M. EST)

National Women's Health Network
514 10th Street, N.W. Suite 400
Washington, DC 20004
(202) 347-1140

National Lesbian and Gay Health Association
Lesbian Health Advocacy Network
1407 S Street, N.W.
Washington, DC 20009
(202) 797-3536

National Black Women's Health Project
1237 Ralph David Abernathy Boulevard, S.W.
Atlanta, GA 30310
(404) 758-9590

National Latina Health Organization
P.O. Box 7567
Oakland, CA 94601
(510) 534-1362

National Asian Women's Health Organization
250 Montgomery Street, Suite 410
San Francisco, CA 94104
(415) 989-9747

Appendix III

WHERE TO GO FOR
HELP WITH SLEEP

If you have any questions about sleep or sleep disorders, please contact us:

New York University Sleep Disorders Center
NYU School of Medicine
462 First Avenue (7N3)
New York, NY 10016
Joyce A. Walsleben, R.N., PhD., Director
David M. Rapoport, M.D., Medical Director
212-263-8423/Fax: 212-562-4677
E-mail: Joyce.Walsleben@med.nyu.edu

Sleep disorders include problems with sleeping, problems with staying awake, and troublesome behavior during sleep. The American Academy of Sleep Medicine is dedicated to maintaining high medical standards in the diagnosis and treatment of these difficulties. Following is a listing of sleep disorders centers and laboratories that have been accredited by and maintain membership in the American Academy of Sleep Medicine. Member centers provide the diagnosis and treatment of all types of sleep-related disorders, and member laboratories (identified with asterisks) specialize only in sleep-related breathing disorders. A current listing may be obtained from the American Academy of Sleep Medicine on the World Wide Web at http://www.aasmnet.org. However, there are many fine sleep centers that are not affiliated with the academy, so if there's no listing near you, seek a referral from your physician.

ALABAMA

Sleep Disorders Laboratory*
Northeast Alabama Regional Medical
Center
400 East 10th Street,
P.O. Box 2208
Anniston, AL 36202
William J. Ferguson, M.D.
D. Larry Cash
256-235-5077/fax: 256-235-5591

**Sleep-Related Breathing Disorders
Lab***
Athens-Limestone Hospital
700 West Market Street
P.O. Box 999
Athens, AL 35612
Andy Jackson
Cherri Walker
256-771-7378/fax: 256-233-9575

Brookwood Sleep Disorders Center
Brookwood Medical Center
2010 Brookwood Medical Center
Drive
Birmingham, AL 35209
Robert C. Doekel, M.D.
B. J. Slonneger, R.P.S.G.T.
205-877-2403/fax: 205-877-1663

**Princeton Sleep/Wake Disorders
Center**
Baptist Medical Center Princeton
701 Princeton Avenue SW
P.O.B. II, Suite 50
Birmingham, AL 35211-1399
Stuart Padove, M.D., Medical Director
Patsy Stanberry, Secretary
*Herb Caillouet, Administrative Vice
President*
Janet Carlisle, C.R.T., CPAP Manager
205-783-7378/fax: 205-783-7386

**Sleep Disorders Center of Alabama,
Inc.**
790 Montclair Road, Suite 200
Birmingham, AL 35213
Vernon Pegram, Ph.D.
Robert C. Doekel, M.D.
205-599-1020/fax: 205-599-1029

Sleep Disorders Lab*
Carraway Methodist Medical Center
1600 Carraway Boulevard
Birmingham, AL 35234
Kurvilla George
Aneshia Williams
205-502-6164/fax: 205-502-5210

Sleep-Wake Disorders Center
University of Alabama at
Birmingham
1713 6th Avenue South
CPM Building, Room 270
Birmingham, AL 35233-0018
Susan Harding, M.D.
Vernon Pegram, Ph.D.
John McBurney, M.D.
*Len Shigley, R.P.S.G.T., Technical
Director*
205-934-7110/fax: 205-934-6870
E-mail: lshigley@uabmc.edu

**Breathing Related Sleep Disorders
Center***
Marshall Medical Center South
601A Corley Avenue, P.O. Box 758
Boaz, AL 35957
Lori Johnson, R.P.S.G.T., Coordinator
Robert Doekel, Jr., M.D.
256-593-1226/fax: 256-840-4702
E-mail: lori.johnson@mmcs.org

Sleep Disorders Center
Cullman Regional Medical Center
1912 Alabama Highway 157
Cullman, AL 35056-1108
*G. Scott Warner, M.D., Medical
    Director*
*Lisa Nelson Barnett, R.P.S.G.T.,
    Administrative Director*
256-737-2140/fax: 256-737-2261

**Decatur General Sleep Disorders
Center**
1201 7th Street, SE
Decatur, AL 35601
Edward M. Turpin, M.D.
Marc A. Hays, R.R.T.
256-340-2558/fax: 256-340-2566

Sleep-Wake Disorders Center
Flowers Hospital
4370 West Main Street,
    P.O. Box 6907
Dothan, AL 36305
Ronald C. Kornegay, R.P.S.G.T.
Ann B. McDowell, M.D.
Alan Purvis, M.D.
David Davis, M.D.
334-793-5000 Ext. 1685/fax: 334-
    615-7213

Thomas Hospital Sleep Services*
Thomas Hospital
188 Hospital Drive, Suite 201
Fairhope, AL 36532
William E. Goetter, M.D., F.C.C.P.
James J. Griffin, M.D.
334-990-1940/fax: 334-990-1941

ECM Sleep Disorders Lab*
Eliza Coffee Memorial Hospital
205 Marengo Street, P.O. Box 818
Florence, AL 35631

Felix Morris, M.D.
Byron Jamerson, R.P.S.G.T.
256-768-9153/fax: 256-740-8524

**Sleep Diagnostics of Northeast
Alabama for Breathing Related
Disorders***
Gadsden Regional Medical Center
1007 Goodyear Avenue
Gadsden, AL 35903
*Denise J. Barton, R.R.T., R.P.S.G.T.,
    Lead Technologist*
*Stephen Coleman, M.D., Medical
    Director*
256-494-4551/fax: 256-494-4602
Web site:
    www.GADSDENREGIONAL.
    COM

**Crestwood Center for Sleep
Disorders**
250 Chateau Drive, Suite 235
Huntsville, AL 35801
Robert A. Serio, M.D.
Richard M. Sneeringer, M.D.
Angela Murdock Beegle, R.P.S.G.T.
256-880-4710/fax: 256-880-4708

Sleep Center at Huntsville Hospital
911 Big Cove
Huntsville, AL 35801
Paul LeGrand, M.D.
*Debra J. Vaughn, M.B.A., R.R.T.,
    R.P.S.G.T.*
256-517-8553/fax: 256-517-8388
E-mail: paull@md.hhsys.org or
    debrav@lab.hhsys.org

Sleep Disorders Center
Mobile Infirmary Medical Center
P.O. Box 2144
Mobile, AL 36652

Robert Dawkins, Ph.D., M.P.H.
Emerson Kerr, B.S., R.R.T.
334-435-5559 or 800-422-2027/
fax: 334-435-5222
E-mail:
rdawkins.eta@worldnet.att.net or
emersonkerr@vhasecure.net

**Southeast Regional Center for
Sleep/Wake Disorders**
Springhill Memorial Hospital
3719 Dauphin Street
Mobile, AL 36608
Lawrence S. Schoen, Ph.D.
334-460-5319/fax: 334-460-5464

**USA Knollwood Sleep Disorders
Center**
University of South Alabama
Knollwood Park Hospital
5644 Girby Road
Mobile, AL 36693-3398
William A. Broughton, M.D.
334-660-5757/fax: 334-660-5254
E-mail: JETBROU@IBM.NET

Sleep Disorders Center
Baptist Medical Center South
2105 East South Boulevard
Montgomery, AL 36116-2498

David P. Franco, M.D.
Tammy Taylor, R.P.S.G.T.
334-286-3252/fax: 334-286-3108

Sleep Disorders Lab*
East Alabama Medical Center
2000 Pepperell Parkway
Opelika, AL 36801-5452
Gina White, R.R.T., R.P.S.G.T.
Steven E. Dekich, M.D.
334-705-2404/fax: 334-705-2403
E-mail: nancy-strickland@eamc.org
Web site: www.eamc.org

Sleep Disorders Lab*
Helen Keller Hospital
P.O. Box 610
Sheffield, AL 35660
Paul Schuler, M.D.
Ronda Hood, R.R.T.
256-386-4191/fax: 256-386-4323
E-mail: rhood@helenkeller.com

Tuscaloosa Clinic Sleep Center
701 University Boulevard East
Tuscaloosa, AL 35401
Richard M. Snow, M.D., F.C.C.P.
205-349-4043/fax: 205-345-0813
E-mail: rmaxsnow@aol.com

ALASKA

Sleep Disorders Center
Providence Alaska Medical Center
3200 Providence Drive
P.O. Box 196604
Anchorage, AK 99519-6604
*Anne H. Morris, M.D., Medical
Director*
*Gerald Trodden, R.P.S.G.T., Clinical
Manager*

907-261-3650/fax: 907-261-4810
E-mail: JTrodden@provak.org

ARIZONA

Samaritan Regional Sleep Disorders Program
Thunderbird Samaritan Medical Center in Glendale
5555 West Thunderbird Road
Glendale, AZ 85306-4622
Bernard E. Levine, M.D.
Stephen Anthony, M.D.
Connie Boker, R.P.S.G.T.
602-588-4800/fax: 602-588-4810

Samaritan Regional Sleep Disorders Program
Desert Samaritan Medical Center
1400 South Dobson Road
Mesa, AZ 85202
Paul Barnard, M.D.
Tom Munzlinger, B.S., R.P.S.G.T.
602-835-3684/fax: 602-835-8788

Samaritan Regional Sleep Disorders Program
Good Samaritan Regional Medical Center
1111 East McDowell Road

Phoenix, AZ 85006
Bernard Levine, M.D.
David Baratz, M.D.
Connie Boker, R.P.S.G.T.
602-239-5815/fax: 602-239-2129
Web site: www.samaritanAZ.com

Sleep Disorders Center at Scottsdale Healthcare
Scottsdale Healthcare Shea
9003 East Shea Boulevard
Scottsdale, AZ 85260
Jeffrey S. Gitt, D.O.
Sharon E. Cichocki, R.P.S.G.T.
480-860-3200/fax: 480-860-3251

Sleep Disorders Center
University of Arizona
1501 North Campbell Avenue
Tucson, AZ 85724
Stuart F. Quan, M.D.
520-694-6112 or 520-626-6115/fax:
520-694-2515
E-mail: squan@sneeze.resp-sci.arizona.edu

ARKANSAS

Sleep Disorders Center
Washington Regional Medical Center
1125 North College Avenue
Fayetteville, AR 72703
David L. Brown, M.D., Director
William A. Rivers, R.P.S.G.T.,
Coordinator
501-713-1272/fax: 501-713-1190

Pediatric Sleep Disorders
Arkansas Children's Hospital
800 Marshall Street
Little Rock, AR 72202-3591

May Griebel, M.D.
Linda Rhodes, E.M.T., R.P.S.G.T.
501-320-1893/fax: 501-320-6878
E-mail: lkr@exchange.ach.uams.edu

Sleep Disorders Center
Baptist Medical Center
9601 I-630, Exit 7
Little Rock, AR 72205-7299
David Davila, M.D.
Buddy Marshall, C.R.T.T., R.P.S.G.T.
501-202-1902/fax: 501-202-1874

E-mail: dgdavila@baptist-health.org
or HLMARSHA@baptist-
health.org
Web site: www.baptist-health.com

CALIFORNIA

Southern California Sleep Disorders Specialists
1101 South Anaheim Boulevard
Anaheim, CA 92805
Clyde Dos Santos, M.D., Medical Director
Deborah Kerr, Director
714-491-1159/fax: 714-563-2865
E-mail: dkerr@vwmc.com
Web site: www.Tenethealth.com/
Westernmedical/

Sleep Center
Mercy San Juan Hospital
6401 Coyle Avenue, Suite 109
Carmichael, CA 95608
Janice K. Herrmann, R.P.S.G.T., M.A.
Richard Stack, M.D.
916-864-5874/fax: 916-864-5870
E-mail: rstack@sma.com

Sleep Disorders Institute
St. Jude Medical Center
1915 Sunny Crest Drive
Fullerton, CA 92835
Louis J. McNabb, M.D.
Justine Petrie, M.D.
Robert Roethe, M.D.
714-446-7240/fax: 714-446-7245

Glendale Adventist Medical Center Sleep Disorders Center
Glendale Adventist Medical Center
1509 Wilson Terrace
Glendale, CA 91206
David A. Thompson, M.D.

Kathy Cavander
818-409-8323/fax: 818-546-5625

Pacific Sleep Medicine Services
La Jolla Center
9834 Genesee Avenue, Suite 328
La Jolla, CA 92037-1223
Milton Erman, M.D.
Stuart Menn, M.D.
858-657-0550/fax: 858-657-0559
E-mail: merman@scripps.edu or
sjmsleepmed@compuserve.com
Web site: www.sleepmedservices.com

Sleep Disorders Center
Grossmont Hospital
P.O. Box 158
La Mesa, CA 91944-0158
Ellie Hoey, R.P.S.G.T.
619-644-4488/fax: 619-644-4021

Loma Linda Sleep Disorders Center
Loma Linda University Community
Medical Center
25333 Barton Road
Loma Linda, CA 92354
Ralph Downey, III, Ph.D.
*Joanne MacQuarrie, R.R.T.,
R.P.S.G.T.*
909-478-6344/fax: 909-478-6343
Web site: www.llu.edu/llumc/sleep

Sleep Disorders Center
Long Beach Memorial Medical
Center
2801 Atlantic Avenue, P.O. Box 1428

Long Beach, CA 90801-1428
Stephen E. Brown, M.D.
Monir Kashani, R.R.T., R.P.S.G.T.,
Technical Coordinator
877-536-3314/fax: 562-933-0201

UCLA Sleep Disorders Center
24-221 CHS, Box 957069
Los Angeles, CA 90095-7069
Frisca Yan-Go, M.D.
310-206-8005/fax: 310-206-3348

Clinical Monitoring Center, Inc.
Sleep Disorders Center
555 Knowles Drive, Suite 218
Los Gatos, CA 95032
Tom Pace, R.P.S.G.T., Clinical
Coordinator
Laughton Miles, M.D., Ph.D.
408-341-2080/fax: 408-341-2088
E-mail: CMC@sleepscape.com
Web site: http://www.sleepscape.com

Mercy Hospital Sleep Laboratory*
Mercy Hospital and Health Services
2740 M Street
Merced, CA 95340
A. Adam Williams, R.R.T., M.B.A.
Sunit Patel, M.D.
209-384-4726/fax: 209-384-4727
E-mail: AWilliams@CHW.edu

Sleep Disorders Institute
27800 Medical Center Road,
   Suite 210
Mission Viejo, CA 92691
Louis McNabb, M.D.
Justine Petrie, M.D.
Robert Roethe, M.D.
Rose Ann Zumstein, R.P.S.G.T.

Sleep Disorders Center
Hoag Presbyterian Memorial
   Hospital
One Hoag Drive, P.O. Box 6100
Newport Beach, CA 92658-6100
Catherine L. Rain, Coordinator
Paul A. Selecky, M.D.
949-760-2070/fax: 949-574-6297
E-mail: crain@hoaghospital.org
Web site: www.hoag.org

Sleep Evaluation Center
Northridge Hospital Medical Center
18300 Roscoe Boulevard
Northridge, CA 91328
Jeremy Cole, M.D.
David Brandes, M.D.
Dennis McGinty, Ph.D.
Ron Szymusiak, Ph.D.
818-885-5344

California Center for Sleep
   Disorders
3012 Summit Street, 5th Floor,
   South Building
Oakland, CA 94609
Jerrold Kram, M.D.
Glenn Roldan, B.S., R.P.S.G.T.
510-834-8333/fax: 510-834-4728
E-mail: sleepsmart@yahoo.com
Web site: www.sleepsmart.com

St. Joseph Hospital Sleep Disorders
   Center
1310 West Stewart Drive, Suite 403
Orange, CA 92868
Sarah Mosko, Ph.D.
714-771-8950/fax: 714-744-8541

Sleep Disorders Center
University of California, Irvine
101 The City Drive, Route 23
Orange, CA 92868
Peter A. Fotinakes, M.D.
714-456-5105/fax: 714-456-7822

Premier Diagnostics, Inc.
1851 Holser Walk, Suite 210
Oxnard, CA 93030
Jerry Harris, R.C.P., R.R.T.
Rebecca Palmieri, R.C.P., R.R.T.,
R.N., B.S.
George Yu, M.D.
805-485-2633/fax: 805-485-6650
Web site: www.sleep-diagnostics.com

Sleep Disorders Center
Huntington Memorial Hospital
100 West California Boulevard
P.O. Box 7013
Pasadena, CA 91109-7013
Steven Lenik, R.P.S.G.T.
Charles A. Anderson, M.D.
Richard A. Shubin, M.D.
626-397-3061/fax: 626-397-3211
E-mail: SLEEPLAB@ix.netcom.com

Sleep Disorders Center
Doctors Medical Center—Pinole
2151 Appian Way
Pinole, CA 94564-2578
Geoffrey Hux, R.P.S.G.T.
Frederick Nachtwey, M.D.
Richard Sankary, M.D.
510-741-2525 or 800-640-9440/
    fax: 510-724-2189
E-mail:
    GEOFFREY.HUX@tenethealth.
    com
Web site: www.tenethealth.com

Sleep Disorders Center
Pomona Valley Hospital Medical
    Center
1798 North Garey Avenue
Pomona, CA 91767
Dennis Nicholson, M.D.
Fares Elghazi, M.D.
Robert Jones, M.D., F.C.C.P.
909-865-9587/fax: 909-865-9969

Center for Sleep Apnea*
Redding Medical Center
2701 Old Eureka Way, Suite 1I
Redding, CA 96001
Everett Trevor, M.D.
Jean Amari-Melancon, R.P.S.G.T.
530-242-6821/fax: 530-242-6421

Sequoia Sleep Disorders Center
Sequoia Health Services
170 Alameda de las Pulgas
Redwood City, CA 94062-2799
J. Al Reichert, R.P.S.G.T.
Bernhard Votteri, M.D., Medical
    Director
650-367-5137/fax: 650-363-5304
E-mail: sleep@sleepscene.com
Web site: http://www.sleepscene.com

Sutter Sleep Disorders Center
650 Howe Avenue, Suite 910
Sacramento, CA 95825
David J. Groza, R.P.S.G.T., R.C.P.,
    E.E.E.
Lydia Wytrzes, M.D.
916-646-3300/fax: 916-646-4603
E-mail: GROZAD@SutterHealth.org

UCDMC Sleep Disorders Center
University of California, Davis,
    Medical Center
2315 Stockton Boulevard,
    Room 5305

Sacramento, CA 95817
Masud Seyal, M.D., Ph.D.
William Bonekat, D.O.
916-734-0256/fax: 916-736-2976

Inland Sleep Center
401 East Highland Avenue, Suite 552
San Bernardino, CA 92404
Sunil Arora, M.D.
909-883-8058/fax: 909-881-4607

Mercy Sleep Disorders Center
Scripps Mercy Hospital
4077 Fifth Avenue
San Diego, CA 92103-2180
Alex Mercandetti, M.D., F.C.C.P.,
*   Medical Director*
Cheryl L. Spinweber, Ph.D., Clinical
*   Director*
619-260-7378/fax: 619-686-3990
E-mail: sleepctr@mercysd.com
Web site: www.scrippshealth.org

San Diego Sleep Disorders Center
1842 Third Avenue
San Diego, CA 92101
Renata Shafor, M.D.
619-235-0248/fax: 619-544-0588
E-mail: shafor@znet.com

Stanford Health Services Sleep
**   Clinic in San Francisco**
3700 California Street
San Francisco, CA 94118
Bruce T. Adornato, M.D.
Christopher R. Brown, M.D.
Rowena Korobkin, M.D.
Alex Clerk, M.D.
Clete Kushida, M.D., Ph.D.
Anstella Robinson, M.D.
Rafael Pelayo, M.D.
415-750-6336/fax: 415-750-6337

UCSF/Stanford Sleep Disorders
**   Center**
University of California, San
   Francisco
1600 Divisadero Street
San Francisco, CA 94115
David M. Claman, M.D.
Kimberly A. Trotter, M.A., R.P.S.G.T.
415-885-7886/fax: 415-885-3650

Sleep Disorders Center of Santa
**   Barbara**
2410 Fletcher Avenue, Suite 201
Santa Barbara, CA 93105
Andrew S. Binder, M.D.
Laurie Laatsch, R.P.S.G.T.
805-898-8845/fax: 805-898-8848

St. John's Medical Plaza Sleep
**   Disorders Center**
1301 Twentieth Street, Suite 370
Santa Monica, CA 90404
Paul B. Haberman, M.D.
310-828-2293/fax: 310-315-0339
E-mail: phaberma@ucla.edu

Sleep Disorders Clinic
Stanford University Medical Center
401 Quarry Road
Stanford, CA 94305
Jed Black, M.D.
650-723-6601/fax: 650-725-8910

Torrance Memorial Medical Center
**   Sleep Disorders Center**
3330 West Lomita Boulevard
Torrance, CA 90505
Lawrence W. Kneisley, M.D.
310-517-4617/fax: 310-784-4869

Sleep Disorders Laboratory*
Kaweah Delta District Hospital
400 West Mineral King Avenue
Visalia, CA 93291

William R. Winn, M.D.
Gregory C. Warner, M.D.
Larry Kellett, B.S., R.C.P.T., Clinical
  Coordinator
559-624-2338/fax: 559-635-4059
E-mail: ikellett@kdhcd.org

West Valley Sleep Disorders Center
7320 Woodlake Avenue, Suite 140
West Hills, CA 91307
Gordon Dowds, M.D., Medical
  Director

Pamela Pierce, Director
818-715-0096/fax: 818-716-1875
E-mail: gordon@dowds.com

Sleep Disorders Center
Woodland Memorial Hospital
1325 Cottonwood Street
Woodland, CA 95695
Richard A. Beyer, M.D.
Marie Kearney, Manager
530-668-2695/fax: 530-662-9174
E-mail: m2kearney@chw.edu

COLORADO

**Sleep Health Center at National
  Jewish Medical Center**
1400 Jackson Street, A200
Denver, CO 80206
Robert D. Ballard, M.D.
303-270-2109/fax: 303-270-2109

Sleep Center of Southern Colorado
Parkview Medical Center
400 West Sixteenth Street
Pueblo, CO 81003
James Pagel, M.D.
Ron Fossceco, R.R.T., R.P.S.G.T.
719-584-4659/fax: 719-584-4929
E-mail: ronf@parkviewmc.com

CONNECTICUT

**Danbury Hospital Sleep Disorders
  Center**
Danbury Hospital
24 Hospital Avenue
Danbury, CT 06810
Arthur Kotch, M.D.
Arthur Spielman, Ph.D.
203-731-8033/fax: 203-731-8628
E-mail: Kotcha@DanHosp.org

Yale Center for Sleep Disorders
Yale University School of Medicine
333 Cedar Street, P.O. Box 208057
New Haven, CT 06520-8057
Vahid Mohsenin, M.D.
203-737-5556/fax: 203-453-0630

E-mail: sleep.disorders@yale.edu
Web site: info.med.yale.edu/
  intmed/sleep

**Gaylord-Wallingford Sleep
  Disorders Laboratory***
Gaylord Hospital
Gaylord Farms Road
Wallingford, CT 06492
Thomas Whelan, R.P.S.G.T.
Vahid Mohsenin, M.D.
203-284-2853/fax: 203-284-2746

DELAWARE

Sleep Disorders Center
Christiana Care Health Systems
4755 Ogletown-Stanton Road
P.O. Box 6001
Newark, DE 19718
John B. Townsend III, M.D.
Thomas C. Mueller, M.D.
Mary Rose Hancock
302-428-4600/fax: 302-733-2533

Sleep Disorders Center
Christiana Care Health Services
Wilmington Hospital
501 West 14th Street
Wilmington, DE 19899
John B. Townsend III, M.D.
Thomas C. Mueller, M.D.
302-428-4600/fax: 302-733-2533
E-mail:
    Hancock.M@christianacare.org

DISTRICT OF COLUMBIA

**Sibley Memorial Hospital Sleep
    Disorders Center**
5255 Loughboro Road, N.W.
Washington, DC 20016
David N. F. Fairbanks, M.D.
Samuel J. Potolicchio, M.D.
202-364-7676/fax: 202-362-9378

Sleep Disorders Center
5 Main Hospital
Georgetown University Hospital
3800 Reservoir Road, N.W.
Washington, D.C. 20007-2197
Marilyn L. Faucette, R.P.S.G.T.
Anne O'Donnell, M.D.
Kenneth Plotkin, M.D.
*Richard E. Waldhorn, M.D., Medical
    Director*
202-784-3610/fax: 202-784-2920

FLORIDA

Boca Raton Sleep Disorders Center
899 Meadows Road, Suite 101
Boca Raton, FL 33486
Natalio J. Chediak, M.D.
Sheila R. Shafer, C.M.A.
561-750-9881/fax: 561-750-9644

**Florida Hospital Celebration Sleep
    Disorders Center**
Florida Hospital
400 Celebration Place
Celebration, FL 34747
Morris T. Bird, M.D.

Robert S. Thornton, M.D.
Martha McNamara
407-303-4002/fax: 407-303-4303

Mayo Sleep Disorders Center
Mayo Clinic Jacksonville
4500 San Pablo Road
Jacksonville, FL 32224
Paul Fredrickson, M.D.
Joseph Kaplan, M.D.
904-953-7287/fax: 904-953-7388

Watson Clinic Sleep Disorders Center
Watson Clinic, LLP
1600 Lakeland Hills Boulevard
P.O. Box 95000
Lakeland, FL 33804-5000
Eberto Pineiro, M.D.
941-680-7627/fax: 941-680-7430

Atlantic Sleep Disorders Center
1401 South Apollo Boulevard, Suite A
Melbourne, FL 32901
Dennis K. King, M.D.
David R. Schneider, R.P.S.G.T.
407-952-5191/fax: 407-952-7262
E-mail: DKingMD@aol.com

Sleep Disorders Center
Mt. Sinai Medical Center
4300 Alton Road
Miami Beach, FL 33140
Alejandro D. Chediak, M.D.
305-674-2613/fax: 305-674-2647

Sleep Disorders Center
Miami Children's Hospital
6125 Southwest Thirty-first Street
Miami, FL 33155
Marcel J. Deray, M.D.
305-669-7136/fax: 305-669-6472
E-mail: Maderay@aol.com

University of Miami School of Medicine
JMH and VA Medical Center Sleep Disorders Center
Department of Neurology (D4-5)
P.O. Box 016960
Miami, FL 33101
Bruce Nolan, M.D.
305-324-3371
E-mail: bnolan@med.miami.edu

Web site:
miami.edu/neurology/centers/sleep.html

Munroe Regional Medical Center Sleep Laboratory*
Munroe Regional Medical Center
131 Southwest Fifteenth Street
Ocala, FL 34473
Keith Tighe, Director
Joy Nunez, Assistant Director
352-351-7385/fax: 352-351-7280

Florida Hospital Sleep Disorders Center
601 East Rollins Avenue
Orlando, FL 32803
Morris T. Bird, M.D.
Robert S. Thornton, M.D.
407-303-1558/fax: 407-303-1775

Orlando Regional Sleep Disorders Center
Orlando Regional Healthcare Systems
23 West Copeland Drive
Orlando, FL 32806
Barry Decker, M.D.
Geri Lockhart, B.S., R.P.S.G.T., R.R.T.
407-649-6869/fax: 407-872-3876
E-mail: geril@orhs.org

Health First Sleep Disorders Center
Palm Bay Community Hospital
1425 Malabar Road, NE, Suite 250
Palm Bay, FL 32907
John Jessup, M.D.
Anna Barker, B.A., R.P.S.G.T.
407-434-8087/fax: 407-434-8496
E-mail: abarker@health-first.org

Sleep Disorders Center
West Florida Regional Medical
  Center
8383 North Davis Highway
Pensacola, FL 32514
Jane Wilkinson, Director
850-494-4850/fax: 850-494-4809

Suncoast Sleep Disorders Center
Charlotte Regional Medical Center
733 East Olympia Avenue
Punta Gorda, FL 33950
Carlos E. Maas, M.D., F.A.C.P.,
  Medical Director
Mary Darling, R.P.S.G.T., Coordinator
941-637-3141/fax: 941-637-3189

Sleep Center
St. Cloud Hospital
2906 Seventeenth Street
St. Cloud, FL 34769
Barry Decker, M.D.
Geri Lockhart
800-523-8144/fax: 407-872-3876

St. Petersburg Sleep Disorders
  Center
Palms of Pasadena Hospital
1501 Pasadena Avenue South
St. Petersburg, FL 33707
Neil T. Feldman, M.D.

813-360-0853 or 800-242-3244 (in
  Florida)

Sleep Disorders Center
Sarasota Memorial Hospital
1700 South Tamiami Trail
Sarasota, FL 34239
Glenn D. Adams, M.D., Medical
  Director
941-917-2525/fax: 941-917-6187

Tallahassee Sleep Disorders Center
1304 Hodges Drive, Suite B
Tallahassee, FL 32308-4613
George F. Slade, M.D.
800-662-4278 ext. 4 or 850-878-
  7271/fax: 850-878-1509
E-mail: N47593@aol.com

Laboratory for Sleep-Related
  Breathing Disorders*
University Community Hospital
3100 East Fletcher Avenue
Tampa, FL 33613
Daniel J. Schwartz, M.D.
David Bollinger, R.P.S.G.T.,
  R.E.E.G.T.
813-979-7410/fax: 813-615-0878
E-mail: DJSCHWARTZ@pol.net
Web site: www.uch.org

GEORGIA

Atlanta Center for Sleep Disorders
303 Parkway Drive, Box 44
Atlanta, GA 30312
Patrick Merrill, R.P.S.G.T.
Francis Buda, M.D.
Jonne Walter, M.D.
Robert Schnapper, M.D.
404-265-3722/fax: 404-265-3833

Sleep Disorders Center
Northside Hospital
5780 Peachtree Dunwoody Road,
  Suite 150
Atlanta, GA 30342
Russell Rosenberg, Ph.D.

John E. Lee, M.D.
David Westerman, M.D.
404-851-8135/fax: 404-252-9946
E-mail: nshsleep@mindspring.com

Sleep Disorders Center of Georgia
5505 Peachtree Dunwoody Road,
    Suite 370
Atlanta, GA 30342
D. Alan Lankford, Ph.D.
James J. Wellman, M.D.
404-257-0080/fax: 404-257-0592

Sleep Disorders Center
Wellstar Cobb Hospital
3950 Austell Road
Austell, GA 30106
Susan T. Keller, Coordinator
Mark Letica, M.D.
Aris Iatridis, M.D., Medical Director
770-732-2250/fax: 770-732-7217

Sleep Disorders Center
DeKalk Medical Center
2665 North Decatur Road, Suite 435
Decatur, GA 30033
Mark T. Pollock, M.D., F.C.C.P.,
    Medical Director
Michael J. Breus, Ph.D., Clinical
    Director
404-294-4018/fax: 404-501-7088

Central Georgia Sleep Disorders
    Center
777 Hemlock Street, Second Floor
P.O. Box 1035
Macon, GA 31202
Charles C. Wells, M.D., Medical
    Director
Todd Jones, Technical Director
912-633-7222/fax: 912-745-5125
E-mail: CGSDC51113@aol.com

Sleep Disorders Center
Wellstar Kennestone Hospital
677 Church Street
Marietta, GA 30060
William Dowdell, M.D.
David Lesch, M.D.
Susan T. Keller, R.P.S.G.T.
770-793-5353/fax: 770-793-5357

Department of Sleep Disorders
    Medicine
Candler Hospital
5353 Reynolds Street
Savannah, GA 31405
James A. Daly III, M.D., Medical
    Director
Pamela Rockett, R.P.S.G.T., R.R.T.
912-692-6673/fax: 912-692-6931
E-mail: RockettP@St.josephs-
    Candler.org

Savannah Sleep Disorders Center at
    St. Joseph's Hospital
No. 1 St. Joseph's Professional Plaza
11706 Mercy Boulevard
Savannah, GA 31419
Anthony M. Costrini, M.D.,
    D.,A.B.S.M.
912-927-5141/fax: 912-921-3380
E-mail: YAWN11706@aol.com

Sleep Disorders Center
Memorial Health Systems
4700 Waters Avenue
Savannah, GA 31403
Herbert F. Sanders, M.D.
Stephen L. Morris, M.D.
912-350-8327/fax: 912-350-7281

HAWAII

**Orchid Isle Sleep Disorders
  Laboratory***
1404 Kilauea Avenue
Hilo, HI 96720
*Gilbert J. Ransley, R.R.T., Technical
  Director*
*John P. Dawson, M.D., M.P.H.,
  Medical Director*
808-935-6105/fax: 808-935-0016

Pulmonary Sleep Disorders Center*
Kuakini Medical Center
347 North Kuakini Street
Honolulu, HI 96817
Edward J. Morgan, M.D.
Sonia Lee-Gushi, R.P.S.G.T., C.R.T.T.
808-547-9119/fax: 808-547-9225
E-mail: sleephi@juno.com
Web site: kuakini.org

**Queen's Medical Center Sleep
  Laboratory***
Queen's Medical Center
1301 Punchbowl Street
Honolulu, HI 96813

Bruce A. G. Soll, M.D.
Jamil Sulieman, M.D.
808-547-4396/fax: 808-537-7830
E-mail: bsoll@queens.org

Sleep Disorders Center of the Pacific
Straub Clinic & Hospital
888 South King Street
Honolulu, HI 96813
James W. Pearce, M.D.
Linda Kapuniai, Dr. P.H.
808-522-4448/fax: 808-522-3048
E-mail: sdcop@aloha.net

**Orchid Isle Sleep Disorders
  Laboratory***
Waimea Town Plaza
64-1061 Mamalahoa Highway 105
Kamuela, HI 96743
*Gilbert J. Ransley, R.R.T., Technical
  Director*
*John P. Dawson, M.D., M.P.H.,
  Medical Director*
808-885-9681/fax: 808-885-1705
E-mail: snoozdoggi@aol.com

IDAHO

**Idaho Sleep Disorders Center—
  Boise**
St. Luke's Regional Medical Center
190 East Bannock Street
Boise, ID 83712
Brett Troyer, M.D.
David K. Merrick, M.D.
Stephen W. Asher, M.D.
Mary R. Gable, R.P.S.G.T.
208-381-2440/fax: 208-381-4341

**Idaho Sleep Disorders Center—
  Nampa**
Mercy Medical Center
1512 Twelfth Avenue Road
Nampa, ID 83686
Brett E. Troyer, M.D.
David K. Merrick, M.D.
Mary R. Gable, R.P.S.G.T.
208-463-5820/fax: 208-463-5775

Idaho Diagnostic Sleep Lab*
526-C Shoup Avenue West
Twin Falls, ID 83301
Ron Fullmer, M.D.
Richard Hammond, M.D.
Brian Fortuin, M.D.

Diana Lincoln-Haye, R.R.T., R.C.P.
Robin Baggett
John Williams, R.P.S.G.T.
208-736-7646/fax: 208-736-1569

ILLINOIS

Center for Sleep and Ventilatory
  Disorders
University of Illinois at Chicago
1740 West Taylor Street, Room 536E,
  M/C 722
Chicago, IL 60612
Deborah E. Sewitch, Ph.D.
Maureen Smith, R.P.S.G.T.
312-996-7708/fax: 312-413-0503
E-mail: dsewitch@uic.edu

Sleep Disorder Service and Research
  Center
Rush–Presbyterian–St. Luke's
  Medical Center
1653 West Congress Parkway
Chicago, IL 60612
Rosalind Cartwright, Ph.D.
312-942-5440/fax: 312-942-8961
E-mail: rcartwri@rush.edu
Web site:
  www.rush.edu/Med/Psych/Sleep.
  html

Sleep Medicine Center
Children's Memorial Hospital
2300 Children's Plaza, Box 43
Chicago, IL 60614-3394
Stephen Sheldon, D.O.
Mark Detrojan, R.P.S.G.T., Team
  Leader

Paul Ocon, R.N., M.P.A.,
  Administrator
773-880-8230/fax: 773-880-6300
E-mail: ssheldon@nwu.edu

Sleep Disorders Center
Northwestern Memorial Hospital
201 East Huron, Galter Seventh
  Floor
Chicago, IL 60611
Phyllis, C. Zee, M.D., Ph.D., Director
Steve Baker, M.D.
Glenn Clark, R.P.S.G.T.
312-926-8120/fax: 312-926-6637
E-mail: pczee@merle.acns.nw.edu or
  gaclark@nmh.org

Sleep Disorders Center
University of Chicago Hospitals
5841 South Maryland, MC2091
Chicago, IL 60637
Jean-Paul Spire, M.D.
Helen Rubeiz, M.D.
773-702-1782/fax: 773-702-7998
E-mail:
  jpspire@neurology.bsd.uchicago.
  edu

Sleep Disorders Center
Alexian Brothers Medical Center
810 Biesterfield Road, Suite 409
Elk Grove Village, IL 60007
Robert W. Hart, M.D.
Clifford A. Massie, Ph.D.
847-981-5926/fax: 847-981-2003

Sleep Disorders Center
Evanston Hospital
2650 Ridge Avenue
Evanston, IL 60201
Richard S. Rosenberg, Ph.D.
847-570-2567/fax: 847-570-2984
E-mail: r-rosenberg@nwu.edu

Sleep Disorders Center
Hinsdale Hospital
120 North Oak Street
Hinsdale, IL 60521
Peter Freebeck, M.D., Medical
  Director
Lisa Paauwe, Manager
630-856-3901/fax: 630-856-3907

Carle Regional Sleep Disorders
  Center/Mattoon Branch
200 Lerna Road South
Mattoon, IL 61938
Daniel Picchietti, M.D.
Donald A. Greeley, M.D.
217-383-3198

Sleep Disorders Center
Lutheran General Hospital
1775 Dempster Street
Parkside Center, Suite B06
Park Ridge, IL 60068
Barry Weber, M.D.
Wayne Rubinstein, M.D.
Lauren Witcoff, M.D.
847-723-7024/fax: 847-723-7369

E-mail:
  webermd@advocatehealth.com

C. Duane Morgan Sleep Disorders
  Center
Methodist Medical Center of Illinois
221 Northeast Glen Oak Avenue
Peoria, IL 61636
Arthur W. Fox, M.D., Medical
  Director
309-672-4966 or 309-671-5136/fax:
  309-673-4117

Sleep Disorders Laboratory*
Rockford Health System
2400 North Rockton Avenue
Rockford, IL 61103
Theodore S. Ingrassia III, M.D.
815-971-5595/fax: 815-971-9894

SIU School of Medicine/Memorial
  Medical Center
Sleep Disorders Center, Memorial
  Medical Center
701 North First
Springfield, IL 62781
Joseph Henkle, M.D.
Steven Todd, R.R.T., R.P.S.G.T.
217-788-4269/fax: 217-788-7057
E-mail: jhenkle@siumed.edu

Carle Regional Sleep Disorders
  Center
Carle Foundation Hospital
611 West Park Street
Urbana, IL 61801-2595
Daniel Picchietti, M.D.
Donald A. Greeley, M.D.
217-383-3364/fax: 217-383-7117

Sleep Disorders Center
Central Du Page Hospital
25 North Winfield Road
Winfield, IL 60190

Robert Hart, M.D.
Linda Klora, R.P.S.G.T.
630-933-6982/fax: 630-933-2745
E-mail: Linda_Klora@cdh.org

INDIANA

Sleep Disorders Center
St. Francis Hospital and Health
  Centers
1500 Albany Street, Suite 1110
Beech Grove, IN 46107
Dianna L. Miller, R.P.S.G.T.
Manfred P. Mueller, M.D., F.C.C.P.
317-783-8144/fax: 317-781-1402

St. Mary's Sleep Disorders Center
St. Mary's Medical Center
3700 Washington Avenue
Evansville, IN 47750
David Cocanower, M.D.
Rebecca N. Dicus
812-485-4960/fax: 812 485-7953

St. Joseph Sleep Disorders Center
St. Joseph Medical Center
700 Broadway
Fort Wayne, IN 46802
James C. Stevens, M.D.
Thomandram Sekar, M.D.
219-425-3552/fax: 219-425-3553

Center for Sleep Disorders
Indiana University School of
  Medicine
550 North University Boulevard,
  Room S450
Indianapolis, IN 46202
Brian H. Foresman, D.O., F.C.C.P.
Richard A. Fiero, M.D.
317-274-2136/fax: 317-274-4224

Methodist Sleep Disorders Center
Clarian Health
I-65 at Twenty-first Street
P.O. Box 1367
Indianapolis, IN 46206-1367
Thomas Sullivan, M.D.
Tom Ehle, Manager
317-929-5706/fax: 317-929-8703

Sleep Disorders Center
St. Vincent Hospital and Health
  Services
8401 Harcourt Road
Indianapolis, IN 46260-0160
Rex McKinney
Thomas Cartwright, M.D.
317-338-2152/fax: 317-338-4917

Sleep/Wake Disorders Center
Community Hospitals of Indianapolis
1500 North Ritter Avenue
Indianapolis, IN 46219
Marvin E. Vollmer, M.D.
317-355-4275/fax: 317-351-2785

Sleep/Wake Disorders Center
Winona Memorial Hospital
3232 North Meridian Street
Indianapolis, IN 46208
Kenneth N. Wiesert, M.D.
317-927-2100/fax: 317-927-2914

Sleep Alertness Center
Lafayette Home Hospital
2400 South Street
Lafayette, IN 47904
Frederick Robinson, M.D.
765-447-6811, ext. 2840

IOWA

Sleep Disorders Center
Mary Greeley Medical Center
1111 Duff Avenue
Ames, IA 50010
Selden Spencer, M.D., Director
Mark Hislop, R.R.T., R.P.S.G.T.
515-239-2353/fax: 515-239-6741
E-mail: SleepLab@MGMC.com

Sleep Disorders Center
Department of Neurology
University of Iowa Hospitals and
   Clinics
Iowa City, IA 52242
Mark Eric Dyken, M.D.
319-356-3813/fax: 319-356-4505
E-mail: mark-dyken@uiowa.edu

KANSAS

Sleep Disorders Center
Hays Medical Center
201 East Seventh Street
Hays, KS 67601
Suzanne Bollig, R.R.T., R.P.S.G.T.,
   R.E.E.G.T.
785-623-5373/fax: 785-623-5377
E-mail: sbollig@haysmed.com

Sleep Disorders Center
Overland Park Regional Medical
   Center
10500 Quivira Road
P.O. Box 15959
Overland Park, KS 66215
Michael W. Anderson, Ph.D.
John B. Nelson, M.D.
913-541-5641/fax: 913-541-5443

Sleep Disorders Center
St. Francis Hospital and Medical
   Center
1700 Southwest Seventh Street
Topeka, KS 66606-1690
Ted W. Daughety, M.D.
David D. Miller, R.P.S.G.T.
785-295-7900
E-mail: SlpCtr@aol.com

Sleep Medicine Center of Kansas
Wichita Clinic
818 North Carriage Parkway
Wichita, KS 67208
Thomas J. Bloxham, M.D.
Robert Hendrickson, R.P.S.G.T.
316-651-2250/fax: 316-685-9391
Web site:
   http://www.wichitaclinic.com

KENTUCKY

**Physicians' Center for Sleep
  Disorders**
Graves-Gilbert Clinic
1555 Campbell Lane
P.O. Box 90025
Bowling Green, KY 42102-9007
Michael Zachek, M.D.
Randall Hansbrough, M.D., Ph.D.
Douglas Thomson, M.D., M.P.H.
502-781-5111/fax: 502-782-4263
E-mail: zachekm@Graves-
  GilbertClinic.com

Sleep Disorders Center
Greenview Regional Hospital
1801 Ashley Circle
Bowling Green, KY 42101
Gul K. Sahetya, M.D.
Steven Zeller, R.P.S.G.T.
502-793-2175/fax: 502-793-2177

Sleep Disorders Center
St. Luke Hospital West
7380 Turfway Road
Florence, KY 41042
Steven Scheer, M.D.
606-525-5347/fax: 606-525-5124
E-mail: barnes@healthall.com

**Sleep Disorder Center of St. Luke
  Hospital**
St. Luke Hospital, Inc.
85 North Grand Avenue
Fort Thomas, KY 41075
Steven Scheer, M.D.
606-572-3535/fax: 606-572-3375
E-mail: barnes@healthall.com

Sleep Apnea Center*
Jennie Stuart Medical Center
320 West Eighteenth Street
Hopkinsville, KY 42240

Manoj H. Majmudar, M.D.
Mark L. Pierce, R.R.T., R.P.S.G.T.
502-887-0410/fax: 502-887-0412

Sleep Center
Samaritan Hospital
310 South Limestone
Lexington, KY 40508
*Barbara Phillips, M.D., M.S.P.H.,
  F.C.C.P.*
Gary King, R.R.T., Director
606-226-7006/fax: 606-226-7008
Web site: www.KYSS.org or
  SamaritanHospital.org

Sleep Disorders Center
St. Joseph's Hospital
One St. Joseph Drive
Lexington, KY 40504
James Thompson, M.D.
Kathryn Hansen, B.S.
606-313-1855/fax: 606-312-3021

Caritas Sleep Apnea Center*
Caritas Medical Center
1850 Bluegrass Avenue
Louisville, KY 40215
Pete Moore, M.D.
William Lacy, M.D.
Richard Baker, M.D.
502-361-6555/fax: 502-361-6554

Sleep Disorders Center
Baptist Hospital East
4000 Kresge Way
Louisville, KY 40207
Kenneth C. Anderson, M.D.
Vasudeva G. Iyer, M.D.
Karen Bell, R.R.T., Director
Marilee Burnside, R.P.S.G.T.
502-896-7612/fax: 502-897-8238
E-mail: Mburnside@BHSI.com

Sleep Disorders Center
Norton Audubon Hospital
One Audubon Plaza Drive
Louisville, KY 40217
Pamela McCullough, A.R.N.P.
David Winslow, M.D.
502-636-7459/fax: 502-636-7474

Sleep Disorders Center
University of Louisville Hospital
530 South Jackson Street
Louisville, KY 40202
Barbara J. Rigdon, R.P.S.G.T.,
  R.E.E.G.T.
Vasudeva G. Iyer, M.D.
Eugene C. Fletcher, M.D.
502-562-3792/fax: 502-562-4632

Sleep Medicine Specialists
1169 Eastern Parkway, Suite 3357
Louisville, KY 40217
David H. Winslow, M.D., Director
Diania Alsager, R.P.S.G.T., Clinical
  Manager
502-454-0755/fax: 502-454-3497

Regional Medical Center Lab for
  Sleep-Related Breathing
  Disorders*
900 Hospital Drive
Madisonville, KY 42431
Thomas Gallo, M.D.
Frank Taylor, M.D.
502-825-5918/fax: 502-825-5159

Diller Regional Sleep Disorders
  Center
Lourdes Hospital
1530 Lone Oak Road

Paducah, KY 42001
James Metcalf, M.D.
Rick Irvan, R.E.E.G.T., R.P.S.G.T.,
  Manager
502-444-2660/fax: 502-444-2661
E-mail: Neurodocs@aol.com or
  rdirvan@lourdes-pad.org

Breathing Disorders Sleep Lab*
Pikeville Methodist Hospital
911 South Bypass Road
Pikeville, KY 41501
Ramanarao V. Mettu, M.D., F.A.C.P.,
  F.C.C.P., Medical Director
Sally Compton, R.R.T., Director
Linda Greer, C.R.T.T., Manager
Kathy Shaunessy, C.O.O.
606-437-3989/fax: 606-437-9649

P.A.C. Sleep Disorders Lab*
Pattie A. Clay Hospital
P.O. Box 1600, 801 Eastern Bypass
Richmond, KY 40475
Rajan Joshi, M.D., F.C.C.P.
Tom Grant
David Broughton
606-625-3334/fax: 606-625-3104

Medical Center Sleep Center
456 Burnley Road
Scottsville, KY 42164
Walter Warren, M.D.
Chris A. Barnett, R.R.T.
270-622-2865/fax: 270-622-2869
Web site:
  www.mcbg.org/scottsville/sleep

LOUISIANA

Red River Sleep Center
501 Medical Center Drive, Suite 330
Alexandria, LA 71301
Paul A. Guillory, M.D.
Renick P. Webb, M.D.
318-443-1684/fax: 318-443-9799

Lourdes Sleep Disorders Center
Our Lady of Lourdes Regional
  Medical Center
611 St. Landry
Lafayette, LA 70506
Christine Soileau, R.P.S.G.T.,
  R.E.E.G.T.
318-289-2858/fax: 318-289-2834

Memorial Medical Center Sleep
  Disorders Center
2700 Napoleon Avenue
New Orleans, LA 70115
Gregory S. Ferriss, M.D.
Li Yu, M.D.
504-896-5652/fax: 504-896-5772
E-mail: gferriss@pol.net

Tulane Sleep Disorders Center
1415 Tulane Avenue
New Orleans, LA 70112
Denise Sharon, Ph.D.
504-588-5231/fax: 504-584-1727

LSU Sleep Disorders Center
Louisiana State University Medical
  Center
P.O. Box 33932
Shreveport, LA 71130-3932
Andrew L. Chesson, Jr., M.D.
318-675-5365/fax: 318-675-4440
E-mail: achess@lsumc.edu

Neurology and Sleep Clinic
2205 East Seventieth Street
Shreveport, LA 71105
Nabil A. Moufarrej, M.D.
Annette Berry, R.P.F.T., R.P.S.G.T.
318-797-1585/fax: 318-797-6077
E-mail: Namouf@worldnet.att.net

NSRMC Sleep Disorders Center
North Shore Regional Medical
  Center
100 Medical Center Drive
Slidell, LA 70461
Anwant Chawla, M.D.
Mary B. Jones, B.S., M.T., R.P.S.G.T.
504-646-5711/fax: 504-646-5013

MAINE

St. Mary's Sleep Disorders
  Laboratory*
St. Mary's Regional Medical Center
97 Campus Avenue
Lewiston, ME 04240
Ralph V. Harder, M.D.
Peter J. Leavitt, R.R.T.
207-777-8959

Maine Institute for Sleep Breathing
  Disorders*
930 Congress Street
Portland, ME 04102
George E. Bokinsky, Jr., M.D.
207-871-4535/fax: 207-871-6005

MARYLAND

**Johns Hopkins Sleep Disorders
Center**
Asthma and Allergy Building,
   Room 4B50
Johns Hopkins Bayview Circle
5501 Hopkins Bayview Circle
Baltimore, MD 21224
Philip L. Smith, M.D.
Alan Schwartz, M.D.
410-550-0571/fax: 410-550-3374

Maryland Sleep Disorders Center
Greater Baltimore Medical Center
6701 North Charles Street,
   Suite 4100
Baltimore, MD 21204-6808
Thomas E. Hobbins, M.D.
410-494-9773/fax: 410-823-6635
E-mail: thobbins@psr.org

Frederick Sleep Disorders Center
Frederick Memorial Hospital
400 West Seventh Street
Frederick, MD 21701
Marc Raphaelson, M.D.

Konrad W. Bakker, M.D.
Garland McDonald
301-698-3802

**Sleep-Breathing Disorders Center of
   Hagerstown***
12821 Oak Hill Avenue
Hagerstown, MD 21742
Abdul Waheed, M.D.
Shaheen Iqbal, M.D.
Johny Alencherry, M.D.
301-733-5971/fax: 301-733-5773

Shady Grove Sleep Disorders Center
14915 Broschart Road, Suite 102
Rockville, MD 20850
Jean Neuenkirch, R.P.S.G.T.
301-251-5905/fax: 301-251-6189

**Washington Adventist Sleep
   Disorders Center**
7525 Carroll Avenue
Takoma Park, MD 20912
Marc Raphaelson, M.D.
Konrad W. Bakker, M.D.
301-891-2594

MASSACHUSETTS

Sleep Disorders Center
Beth Israel Deaconess Medical
   Center
330 Brookline Avenue, KS430
Boston, MA 02215
Jean K. Matheson, M.D.
Janet Mullington, Ph.D.
617-667-3237/fax: 617-975-5506
E-mail:
   jmatheso@caregroup.harvard.edu

Sleep Disorders Center
Lahey Clinic
41 Mall Road
Burlington, MA 01805
Paul T. Gross, M.D.
David A. Neumeyer, M.D.
Susan M. Dignan, R.P.S.G.T.
781-744-8251/fax: 781-744-5243
E-mail: Susan.M.Dignan@Lahey.org

Sleep Disorders Institute of Central New England
St. Vincent Hospital
25 Winthrop Street
Worcester, MA 01604

Jayant G. Phadke, M.D.
508-798-6066 (office) or
   508-798-1485 (lab)
fax: 508-798-6373

MICHIGAN

Sleep Disorders Center
St. Joseph Mercy Hospital
P.O. Box 995
Ann Arbor, MI 48106
Thomas R. Gravelyn, M.D.
Sharon S. Potoczak, R.P.S.G.T.
734-712-4651/fax: 734-712-2967

Sleep Disorders Center
University of Michigan Hospitals
1500 East Medical Center Drive
UH8D 8702, Box 0117
Ann Arbor, MI 48109-0115
Brenda Livingston, Coordinator
Michael S. Aldrich, M.D.
Ronald Chervin, M.D.
Beth Malow, M.D.
Alon Avidan, M.D.
734-936-9068/fax: 734-936-5377

Sleep Disorders Center
Bay Medical Center
1900 Columbus Avenue
Bay City, MI 48708
John M. Buday, M.D.
Mary K. Taylor, R.P.S.G.T., R.R.T.
517-894-3332/fax: 517-894-6114

Sleep Disorders Center
Sinai-Grace Hospital
6071 West Outer Drive
Detroit, MI 48235
313-966-3088/fax: 313-966-1250

Sleep Disorders Center at Hutzel Hospital
Hutzel Hospital
4707 St. Antoine, 1 Center
Detroit, MI 48201
James A. Rowley, M.D.
David Calahan, R.R.T.
313-745-9009/fax: 313-745-8725
E-mail: jrowley@intmed.wayne.edu

Sleep/Wake Disorders Laboratory (127B)
VA Medical Center
4646 John R. Street
Detroit, MI 48201-1916
Sheldon Kapen, M.D.
M. Safwan Badr, M.D.
Greg Koshorek
313-576-3663/fax: 313-576-1122
E-mail: kapen.sheldon@allen-
   park.va.gov

West Michigan Sleep Disorders Center
Butterworth Hospital
100 Michigan Street, NE
Grand Rapids, MI 49503
Lee Marmion, M.D.
Ronald Van Drunen, R.P.S.G.T.
616-391-3759/fax: 616-391-3052

Sleep Disorders Center
Borgess Medical Center
1521 Gull Road
Kalamazoo, MI 49001

Sue Cammarata, M.D.
Thomas Wittenberg, R.R.T.
Sheri Dillon, R.R.T.
616-226-7081/fax: 616-226-6909

Ingham Regional Medical Center
Sleep/Wake Center
2025 South Washington Avenue,
   Suite 300
Lansing, MI 48910-0817
Pamela Minkley, R.R.T., R.P.S.G.T.
Gauresh Kashyap, M.D., F.A.C.P.,
   F.C.C.P.
517-372-6444/fax: 517-372-6440
E-mail:
   pam.minkley@worldnet.att.net

Sparrow Sleep Center
Sparrow Hospital
1215 East Michigan Avenue
P.O. Box 30480
Lansing, MI 48909-7980
Alan M. Atkinson, D.O.
David K. Young, D.O.
517-364-5370/fax: 517-364-5373

Sleep and Respiratory Associates of
   Michigan
28200 Franklin Road
Southfield, MI 48034
Harvey W. Organek, M.D.
248-350-2722/fax: 248-350-0154

Munson Sleep Disorders Center
Munson Medical Center
1105 Sixth Street, MPB Suite 307
Traverse City, MI 49684-2386
David A. Walker, D.O., F.C.C.P.,
   Medical Director
Leon R. Olewinski, R.R.T., Director
Marcia Rinal, C.R.T.T., R.P.S.G.T.,
   Manager
800-358-9641 or 616-935-6600/fax:
   616-935-6610
E-mail: mrinal@mhc.net

Sleep Disorders Institute
44199 Dequindre, Suite 311
Troy, MI 48098
R. Bart Sangal, M.D.
248-879-0707/fax: 248-879-2704

MINNESOTA

Duluth Regional Sleep Disorders
   Center
St. Mary's Duluth Clinic Health
   System
407 East Third Street
Duluth, MN 55805
Peter K. Franklin, M.D.
Paul J. Windberg, M.D.
Mary Carlson, R.P.S.G.T.
218-726-4692/fax: 218-726-4083
E-mail: mcarlson@smdc.org

Fairview Sleep Center
Fairview Southdale Hospital
6401 France Avenue South
Edina, MN 55435
John E. Trusheim, M.D.
612-924-5053/fax: 612-924-5994
E-mail: cmunger1@fairview.org

Minnesota Regional Sleep Disorders
   Center, No. 867B
Hennepin County Medical Center
701 Park Avenue South
Minneapolis, MN 55415

Mark Mahowald, M.D.
612-347-6288/fax: 612-904-4207
E-mail:
  mahow002@maroon.tc.umn.edu

Sleep Disorders Center
Abbott Northwestern Hospital
800 East Twenty-eighth Street at
  Chicago Avenue
Minneapolis, MN 55407
Wilfred A. Corson, M.D.
612-863-4516/fax: 612-863-2837
Web site: www.mnsleep.com

Mayo Sleep Disorders Center
Mayo Clinic
200 First Street, SW
Rochester, MN 55905
Peter Hauri, Ph.D.

John W. Shepard, Jr., M.D.
507-266-8900/fax: 507-266-7772
E-mail: hauri.peter@mayo.edu

Sleep Disorders Center
Methodist Hospital
6500 Excelsior Boulevard
St. Louis Park, MN 55426
Barb Feider, R.P.S.G.T.
Salim Kathawalla, M.D.
612-993-6083/fax: 612-993-7026

Health East Sleep Care
St. Joseph's Hospital
69 West Exchange Street
St. Paul, MN 55102
Thomas Mulrooney, M.D.
651-232-3682/fax: 651-291-2932

MISSISSIPPI

Sleep Disorders Center
Memorial Hospital at Gulfport
P.O. Box 1810
Gulfport, MS 39501
Sydney Smith, M.D.
228-865-3152/fax: 228-865-3259

Sleep Disorders Center
Forrest General Hospital
6051 Highway 49, P.O. Box 16389
Hattiesburg, MS 39404-6389
Geoffrey B. Hartwig, M.D.
John R. Harsh, Ph.D.
Dennis Kramer
601-288-1994 or 800-280-8520/
  fax: 601-288-1999
E-mail: gblount@forrestgeneral.com
Web site: www.forrestgeneral.com/
  Sleepdisorders.htm

**Sleep Disorders Center and Division
  of Sleep Medicine**
University of Mississippi Medical
  Center
2500 North State Street
Jackson, MS 39216-4505
*Howard Roffwarg, M.D., D.,A.B.S.M.,
  Director*
*Alp Sinan Baran, M.D., D.,A.B.S.M.,
  Medical Director*
*Allen Richert, M.D., D.,A.B.S.M.,
  Staff Specialist*
601-984-4820/fax: 601-984-5885
E-mail: ASBARAN@POL.NET

MISSOURI

**Unity Sleep Medicine and Research
    Center**
St. Luke's Hospital
232 South Woods Mill Road
Chesterfield, MO 63017
James K. Walsh, Ph.D.
Gihan Kader, M.D.
314-205-6030/fax: 314-205-6025
E-mail: jkw@stlo.smhs.com or
    gak@stlo.smhs.com

**University of Missouri Sleep
    Disorders Center**
M-741 Neurology, University
    Hospital and Clinics
One Hospital Drive
Columbia, MO 65212
Pradeep Sahota, M.D.
573-884-7533 or 800-233-7533/
    fax: 573-884-4785
E-mail: sahotap@health.missouri.edu

Sleep Disorders Center
Research Medical Center
2316 East Meyer Boulevard
Kansas City, MO 64132-1199
Jon D. Magee, Ph.D.
816-276-4334/fax: 816-276-3488

Sleep Disorders Center
St. Luke's Hospital
4400 Wornall Road
Kansas City, MO 64111
Ann M. Romaker, M.D.
816-932-3207/fax: 816-932-3383
E-mail: ecook@saint-lukes.org

**Cox Regional Sleep Disorders
    Center**
3800 South National Avenue,
    Suite LL 150

Springfield, MO 65807
Edward Gwin, M.D.
417-269-5575/fax: 417-269-5578

St. John's Sleep Disorders Center
St. John's Regional Health Center
1235 East Cherokee
Springfield, MO 65804
John Brabson, M.D., Medical Director
Terry M. Yarnell, R.E.E.G.T.,
    R.C.P.T., Administrative Director
417-885-5464/fax: 417-885-5465

**St. Joseph Health Center Sleep
    Disorders Laboratory***
St. Joseph Health Center
300 First Capitol Drive
St. Charles, MO 63301
Thomas M. Siler, M.D.
Susan Townsley, R.P.S.G.T.,
    Laboratory Coordinator
636-947-5165/fax: 636-947-5164
E-mail: thomas.siler.md@ssmhc.com
Web site: www.ssmhc.com

**Sleep Disorders and Research
    Center**
Forest Park Hospital of Tenet Health
    System
6150 Oakland Avenue
St. Louis, MO 63139
Sidney D. Nau, Ph.D.
Korgi V. Hegde, M.D.
314-768-3100/fax: 314-768-3594
E-mail: sid.nau@tenethealth.com

Sleep/Wake Disorders Center
SLU Care, Health Services Division
    of Saint Louis University
1221 South Grand Boulevard

St. Louis, MO 63104
Shashidhar M. Shettar, M.D.
314-577-8705/fax: 314-664-7248
E-mail: shettars@slu.edu

MONTANA

Sleep Center at St. Vincent Hospital
St. Vincent Hospital and Health
   Center
1233 North Thirtieth Street
Billings, MT 59101
William C. Kohler, M.D.
Karen Y. Allen, C.R.T.T., R.P.S.G.T.
406-238-6815/fax: 406-238-6262
E-mail: wkohler@svhhc.org or
   kallen@svhhc.org

Sleep Disorders Center
Deaconess Billings Clinic
2800 Tenth Avenue North
P.O. Box 37000
Billings, MT 59107

Terry Padgett, R.P.S.G.T., R.R.T.
Robert K. Merchant, M.D.
406-657-4075/fax: 406-657-4717
E-mail: rpsgt1@aol.com
Web site: www.billingsclinic.org

St. Patrick Hospital Sleep Center
St. Patrick Hospital
500 West Broadway
Missoula, MT 59802
Stephen F. Johnson, M.D.
Richard B. Wall, R.E.E.G.T.
406-329-5650/fax: 406-329-5605
E-mail: Wall@saintpatrick.org
Web site: www.saintpatrick.org

NEBRASKA

Adult and Pediatric Sleep Related
   Breathing Disorders Laboratory*
Bryan LGH Medical Center East
1600 South 48th Street
Lincoln, NE 68506
Debra Bailey, R.N., Clinical Manager
William M. Johnson, M.D., Medical
   Director
402-481-3950/fax: 402-481-8374
E-mail: dbailey@bryanlgh.org

Great Plains Regional Sleep
   Physiology Center
Bryan LGH Medical Center West
2300 South 16th Street
Lincoln, NE 68502
Timothy R. Lieske, M.D.
Leigh Heithoff, R.P.S.G.T., R.E.E.G.T.

402-481-5338/fax: 402-481-5380
E-mail: leigh.heithoff@bryanlgh.org

Sleep Disorders Center
Methodist/Richard Young Hospital
2566 St. Mary's Avenue
Omaha, NE 68105
Robert J. Ellingson, Ph.D., M.D.
402-354-6305 or 402-354-6309/
   fax: 402-354-6334

Sleep Disorders Center
Nebraska Health System
987546 Nebraska Medical Center
Omaha, NE 68198-7546
Carie L. Smith, R.R.T., R.P.S.G.T.
Stephen B. Smith, M.D.
402-552-2286/fax: 402-552-2057

NEVADA

Mountain Medical Sleep Disorders Center
Mountain Medical Associates, Inc.
710 West Washington Street
Carson City, NV 89703-3826
Robert L. McDonald, M.D.
John T. Zimmerman, Ph.D.
775-882-2106 or 775-882-4139/
    fax: 775-882-0838
E-mail: dzimmer889@aol.com

Sleep Clinic of Nevada at St. Rose Dominican Hospital
102 East Lake Mead Drive
Henderson, NV 89105
John F. Pinto, M.D.
Darlene Steljes, CEO
702-893-0020/fax: 702-893-0025

Sleep Clinic of Nevada
1012 East Sahara Avenue
Las Vegas, NV 89104
Darlene Steljes, CEO
702-893-0020/fax: 702-893-0025

Washoe Sleep Disorders Center and Sleep Laboratory
Washoe Professional Building and
    Washoe Medical Center
Sleep Management, Inc., EYE-COM, Inc.
75 Pringle Way, Suite 701
Reno, NV 89502
William C. Torch, M.D., M.S.
Paul Binks, Ph.D.
John T. Zimmerman, Ph.D.
775-328-4700/fax: 775-329-2715

NEW HAMPSHIRE

Sleep Disorders Center
Dartmouth-Hitchcock Medical
    Center
One Medical Center Drive
Lebanon, NH 03756

Michael Sateia, M.D.
603-650-7534/fax: 603-650-7820
E-mail:
    sleep.disorders.center@dartmouth.edu

NEW JERSEY

SleepCare Center of Cherry Hill
457 Haddonfield Road, Suite 520
Cherry Hill, NJ 08002
James La Russo, CEO
John D. Miladin, President, COO
Kathleen L. Ryan, M.D., F.C.C.P., F.A.C.P.
800-753-3779/fax: 609-662-5187
E-mail: flajack@aol.com
Web site: sleepcarecenter.com

Institute for Sleep/Wake Disorders
Hackensack University Medical
    Center
30 Prospect Avenue
Hackensack, NJ 07601
Hormoz Ashtyani, M.D.
Sue Zafarlotfi, Ph.D.
201-996-3732/fax: 201-498-1163

Sleep Disorder Center
Morristown Memorial Hospital
95 Mount Kemble Avenue
Morristown, NJ 07962
Robert A. Capone, M.D., F.C.C.P.
Pamela Wolfsie, R.P.S.G.T.
973-971-4567/fax: 973-290-7620
Web site: www.atlantichealth.org

SleepCare
Virtua Health
175 Madison Avenue
Mount Holly, NJ 08060
Kathleen L. Ryan, M.D.
John D. Miladin
800-753-3779/fax: 609-662-5187
E-mail: flajack@aol.com
Web site: sleepcarecenter.com

Comprehensive Sleep Disorders Center
Robert Wood Johnson University
    Hospital/UMDNJ
Robert Wood Johnson Medical
    School
One Robert Wood Johnson Place
P.O. Box 2601
New Brunswick, NJ 08903-2601
Richard A. Parisi, M.D.
Raymond Rosen, Ph.D.
732-937-8683/fax: 732-418-8448

Sleep Disorders Center
Newark Beth Israel Medical Center
201 Lyons Avenue
Newark, NJ 07112

Monroe Karetzky, M.D.
973-926-6668/fax: 973-923-6672
E-mail: MKARETZK@sbhcs.com
Web site: www.njsleephelp.com

Mercer Sleep Disorders Center
Capital Health System
446 Bellevue Avenue
Trenton, NJ 08607
Debra DeLuca, M.D.
Rita Brooks, R.E.E.G./E.P.T.,
    R.P.S.G.T., C.N.I.M.
609-394-4167/fax: 609-394-4352
E-mail: Rbrooks@chsnj.org

Snoring and Sleep Apnea Center*
Capital Health System
750 Brunswick Avenue
Trenton, NJ 08638
Marcella Frank, D.O.
Rita Brooks, R.E.E.G./E.P.T.,
    R.P.S.G.T., C.N.I.M.
609-278-6990/fax: 609-278-6982
E-mail: Rbrooks@chsnj.org

Sleep Disorders Center of New Jersey
2253 South Avenue, Suite 7
Westfield, NJ 07090
David S. Goldstein, M.D.
Michael Lahey, R.P.S.G.T.
908-789-4244/fax: 908-789-2716

NEW MEXICO

**New Mexico Center for Sleep
  Medicine**
Lovelace Health Systems
4700 Jefferson, NE
Albuquerque, NM 87110
Lee K. Brown, M.D., Medical Director
*Nancy L. Polnaszek, Director of
  Medical Specialties*
505-872-6000/fax: 505-872-6003
E-mail: nlpoln@lovelace.com
Web site: www.lovelace.com

**University Hospital Sleep Disorders
  Center**
4775 Indian School Road, NE,
  Suite 307
Albuquerque, NM 87110
Rose Mills
Barry Krakow, M.D.
505-272-6101/fax: 505-272-6112

NEW YORK

**Capital Region Sleep/Wake
  Disorders Center**
St. Peter's Hospital
Pine West Plaza, No. 1, Washington
  Avenue Extension
Albany, NY 12205
Aaron E. Sher, M.D.
Paul B. Glovinsky, Ph.D.
518-464-9999/fax: 518-464-9650
E-mail: sleep@mercycare.com

Sleep/Wake Disorders Center
Montefiore Medical Center
111 East 210th Street
Bronx, NY 10467
Michael J. Thorpy, M.D.
718-920-4841/fax: 718-798-4352
E-mail: Thorpy@aecom.yu.edu
Web site:
  www.cloud9.net/~thorpy/mmc/

**Bassett Healthcare Sleep Disorders
  Center**
Bassett Healthcare
One Atwell Road

Cooperstown, NY 13326
Lee C. Edmonds, M.D.
Robert C. Reese, R.R.T., R.P.S.G.T.
607-547-6979/fax: 607-547-6906
E-mail: reesere@hotmail.com
Web site: www.bassetthealthcare.org

**St. Joseph's Hospital Sleep
  Disorders Center**
St. Joseph's Hospital
555 East Market Street
Elmira, NY 14902
Kathleen R. Reilly, B.S., R.R.T.
Paula Cook, R.P.S.G.T., R.R.T.
607-737-7008/fax: 607-737-1522

**Parkway Hospital Sleep Disorders
  Center**
Parkway Hospital
70-35 113th Street
Forest Hills, NY 11375
Jang B. S. Chadha, M.D.
718-990-4590/fax: 718-268-6110
E-mail: info@phsdc.com
Web site: www.phsdc.com

Sleep Disorders Center
Winthrop-University Hospital
222 Station Plaza North
Mineola, NY 11501
Michael Weinstein, M.D.
Maritza Groth, M.D., F.C.C.P.
Claude Albertario, R.P.S.G.T.
516-663-3907/fax: 516-663-4788
E-mail: mweinstein@winthrop.org

Sleep-Wake Disorders Center
Long Island Jewish Medical Center
270-05 76th Avenue
New Hyde Park, NY 11042
Harly Greenberg, M.D.
Jane Luchsinger, M.S.
718-470-7058/fax: 718-470-7058
E-mail: greenber@lij.edu

Sleep Disorders Center
Columbia-Presbyterian Medical
    Center
161 Fort Washington Avenue
New York, NY 10032
Neil B. Kavey, M.D.
212-305-1860 or 914-948-0400/
    fax: 212-305-5496
E-mail: nbk1@columbia.edu

Sleep Disorders Institute
1090 Amsterdam Avenue
New York, NY 10025
Gary K. Zammit, Ph.D.
212-523-1700 or 888-753-3769/
    fax: 212-523-1704
E-mail: gzammit@slrhc.org
Web site: www.sleepny.com

Sleep-Wake Disorders Center
New York Presbyterian Hospital,
    Cornell Campus
520 East 70th Street
New York, NY 10021

Gabriele M. Barthlen, M.D.
Daniel Wagner, M.D.
Margaret Moline, Ph.D.
212-746-2623/fax: 212-746-8984

Sleep Disorders Center of Rochester
2110 Clinton Avenue South
Rochester, NY 14618
Donald W. Greenblatt, M.D.
716-442-4141/fax: 716-442-6259

Sleep Apnea Center*
Staten Island University Hospital
375 Sequine Avenue
Staten Island, NY 10309
R. Ciccone, M.D., Medical Director
T. Kilkenny, D.O., Associate Medical
    Director
Nicholas Caruselle, Administrator
Steve Grenard, R.R.T., Program
    Director
718-226-2332/fax: 718-226-2735
E-mail: sgrenard@siuh.edu

Sleep Center
Community General Hospital
Broad Road
Syracuse, NY 13215
Robert E. Westlake, M.D.
Antonio Culebras, M.D.
Bruce D. Hall, R.P.S.G.T., R.R.T.
315-492-5877/fax: 315-492-5521
Web site: www.cgh.org

Sleep Laboratory*
St. Joseph's Hospital Health Center
945 East Genesee Street, Suite 300
Syracuse, NY 13210
Edward T. Downing, M.D.
Stephen F. Swierczek, R.P.S.G.T.
315-475-3379/fax: 315-475-5077
Web site: www.sjhsyr.org

**Mohawk Valley Sleep Disorders
Center**
St. Elizabeth Medical Center
2209 Genesee Street
Utica, NY 13501
Steven A. Levine, D.O., F.C.C.P.
Mark Cassidy, R.P.S.G.T.
315-734-3484/fax: 315-734-3494
E-mail: mvsdc@stemc.org

**Sleep Disorders Center—White
Plains**
Columbia-Presbyterian Medical
Center
185 Maple Avenue
White Plains, NY 10601

Neil B. Kavey, M.D.
914-948-0400/fax: 212-305-5496
E-mail: nbk1@columbia.edu

Sleep-Wake Disorders Center
New York Presbyterian Hospital—
Cornell Campus
21 Bloomingdale Road
White Plains, NY 10605
*Daniel R. Wagner, M.D., Medical
Director*
Margaret L. Moline, Ph.D., Director
914-997-5751/fax: 914-682-6911
E-mail:
    dwagner@mail.med.cornell.edu or
    mmoline@mail.med.cornell.edu

NORTH CAROLINA

Mission/St. Joseph's Sleep Center
445 Biltmore Avenue, Suite 404
Asheville, NC 28801
Charles O'Cain, M.D.
James McCarrick, M.D.
Jean C. Hardy, R.P.S.G.T.
828-258-6701/fax: 828-258-6702

Carolinas Sleep Services
Mercy Hospital South
16028 Park Road
Charlotte, NC 28210
Mindy B. Cetel, M.D.
Michael Stolzenbach, R.P.S.G.T.
704-543-2213/fax: 704-341-2755

Carolinas Sleep Services
University Hospital
8800 North Tyron Street
P.O. Box 560727
Charlotte, NC 28256
*Mindy B. Cetel, M.D., Medical
Director*

*Michael Stolzenbach, R.P.S.G.T.,
Manager*
704-548-5855 and 877-
    2SLEEPEZ/fax: 704-548-5891

Sleep Disorders Center
Moses Cone Health System
1200 North Elm Street
Greensboro, NC 27401-1020
Clinton D. Young, M.D.
Reggie Whitsett, R.P.S.G.T.
336-832-7406/fax: 336-832-8649

Sleep Medicine Center of Salisbury
911 West Henderson Street,
    Suite L30
Salisbury, NC 28144
Dennis L. Hill, M.D.
Sharon Leach, R.P.S.G.T.
704-637-1533/fax: 704-637-0470
E-mail: hill@2sleepy.com

Sleep Disorders Center
North Carolina Baptist Hospital
Wake Forest University School of
    Medicine
Medical Center Boulevard
Winston-Salem, NC 27157
W. Vaughn McCall, M.D.
Linda Quinlivan, R.P.S.G.T.
336-716-5288/fax: 336-716-9742
E-mail: vmcall@wfubmc.edu or
    lindaq@wfubmc.edu

Web site: www.wfubmc.edu or
    www.wfubmc.edu/neurology/
    department/diagneur.html

Summit Sleep Disorders Center
160 Charlois Boulevard
Winston-Salem, NC 27103
J. Baldwin Smith III, M.D.
Richard Doud Bey, M.D.
336-765-9431/fax: 336-765-4889
E-mail: minnie@netunlimited.net

NORTH DAKOTA
No Accredited Member Centers

OHIO

Cincinnati Regional Sleep Centers
2123 Auburn Avenue, Suite 322
Cincinnati, OH 45219
Bruce C. Corser, M.D.
Joseph W. Zompero, R.P.S.G.T.
513-721-4680/fax: 513-721-1036
Web site: www.crsc.com

**Cincinnati Regional Sleep Centers—
    West**
5049 Crookshank Road, Suite G-3
Cincinnati, OH 45238
Bruce Corser, M.D.
James Armitage, M.D.
Joseph W. Zompero, R.P.S.G.T.
513-347-0220/fax: 513-347-5173

**Sleep Disorders Centers of Greater
    Cincinnati**
TriHealth Hospitals
619 Oak Street
Cincinnati, OH 45206
Virgil Wooten, M.D.
513-569-6320/fax: 513-569-5495

E-mail: virgil_wooten@trihealth.com
Web site: www.trihealth.org

Tri-State Sleep Disorders Center
1275 East Kemper Road
Cincinnati, OH 45246
Martin B. Scharf, Ph.D.
513-671-3101/fax: 513-671-4159
E-mail: SleepSatl@aol.com

**PMA Cardiopulmonary Sleep
    Laboratory***
Pulmonary Medicine Associates, Inc.
15805 Puritas Avenue
Cleveland, OH 44135
Paul C. Venizelos, M.D., F.C.C.P.
Babu M. Eapen, M.D., F.C.C.P.
Petra Podmore, R.P.S.G.T.,
    R.E.E.G.T.
216-267-5933/fax: 216-267-5133

Sleep Disorders Center
Cleveland Clinic Foundation
9500 Euclid Avenue, Desk S-51
Cleveland, OH 44195
Dudley S. Dinner, M.D.
216-444-2165/fax: 216-445-4378

University Hospitals Sleep Center
University Hospitals of Cleveland
Department of Neurology
11100 Euclid Avenue
Cleveland, OH 44106
Carl Rosenberg, M.D., M.B.A.
Lucica Buzoianu
216-844-1301/fax: 216-844-8753

Regional Sleep Disorder Center
Columbus Community Hospital
1430 South High Street
Columbus, OH 43207
Allen Nicholson, Clinical Coordinator
Robert W. Clark, M.D., Medical
    Director
614-437-7800/fax: 614-437-7008
E-mail: flamenco@netexp.net
Web site: www.thesleepsite.com

Sleep Disorders Center
Ohio State University Medical Center
Rhodes Hall, S1039
410 West Tenth Avenue
Columbus, OH 43210-1228
Anthony Brooks
Charles P. Pollak, M.D.
614-293-8296/fax: 614-293-4506

Samaritan North Sleep Center*
9000 North Main Street, Suite 225
Dayton, OH 45415
Rajesh C. Patel, M.D., F.C.C.P.,
    Medical Director
Joyce E. Gray, Manager

937-567-6180/fax: 937-567-6187
E-mail: Jgray@SHP_Dayton.org

Sleep Disorders Center
Kettering Medical Center
3535 Southern Boulevard
Dayton, OH 45429-1295
Donna Arand, Ph.D.
937-296-7805/fax: 937-296-7821
E-mail:
    Donna_Arand@Ketthealth.com

Center for Sleep and Wake
    Disorders
Miami Valley Hospital
One Wyoming Street, Suite G-200
Dayton, OH 45409
James Graham, M.D.
Kevin Huban, Psy.D.
937-208-2515

Marymount Hospital Sleep
    Disorders Center
Marymount Hospital
12300 McCracken Road
Garfield Heights, OH 44125
Raymond J. Salomone, M.D.
A. Romeo Craciun, M.D.
Gary L. Foreman, B.S. R.R.T., R.C.P.
216-587-8151/fax: 216-587-8857
E-mail: gforeman@marymount.org

St. Rita's Sleep Disorders Lab
St. Rita's Medical Center
730 West Market Street
Lima, OH 45801
Jeffrey E. Godwin, M.D., R.Ph.,
    F.C.C.P.
Mary L. Reed
419-226-9397/fax: 419-226-9535
E-mail: mreed@health-partners.org

Sleep Disorders Center
St. Luke's Hospital
5901 Monclova
Maumee, OH 43537
Thomas Calderon, M.D.
Marty Ensman
419-897-8490/fax: 419-897-8491

Meridia Sleep Disorders Center
Meridia-Cleveland Clinic Health
   System
6780 Mayfield Road
Mayfield Heights, OH 44124
Daniel W. Sutton, B.S., R.R.T., R.C.P.
Raymond Salomone, M.D.
Eva Hu-Whittemore, M.D.
440-646-8090/fax: 440-460-2805

Ohio Sleep Disorders Center
150 Springside Drive
Montrose, OH 44333
Jose Rafecas, M.D.
Frankie Roman, M.D.
Larry Sattis, M.D.
330-670-1290/fax: 330-670-1292
E-mail: Green@ohiosleep.com
Web site: www.ohiosleep.com

Sleep Improvement Lab
Mercy Hospital of Tiffin
485 West Market Street
Tiffin, OH 44883

Vicki Edgington, R.R.T., C.P.F.T.,
   R.C.P.
419-448-7666/fax: 419-448-7669
E-mail: vicki_edgington@mhsnr.org

Northwest Ohio Sleep Disorders
   Center
Toledo Hospital
Harris-McIntosh Tower,
   Second Floor
2142 North Cove Boulevard
Toledo, OH 43606
Pam Lang, R.P.S.G.T.
Frank O. Horton III, M.D.
419-471-5629/fax: 419-479-6954

Sleep Disorders Center
St. Vincent Medical Center
3829 Woodley, Suite 1
Toledo, OH 43606
Michael J. Neeb, Ph.D.
419-251-0570/fax: 419-251-0574

Sleep Disorders Center
Genesis Health Care System
Bethesda Hospital
2951 Maple Avenue
Zanesville, OH 43701
Roger J. Balogh, M.D.
Thomas E. Rojewski, M.D.
Robert J. Thompson, M.D.
740-454-4725/fax: 740-450-6168

OKLAHOMA

Sleep Disorders Center of Oklahoma
Integris Health
4401 South Western Avenue
Oklahoma City, OK 73109
Jonathan R. L. Schwartz, M.D.

Elliott R. Schwartz, D.O.
Chris A. Veit, M.S.W., R.P.S.G.T.
405-636-7700/fax: 405-636-7531
E-mail: veitca@integris-health.com
Web site: www.integris-health.com

OREGON

Sleep Disorders Center
Sacred Heart Medical Center
1255 Hilyard Street, P.O. Box 10905
Eugene, OR 97440
Connie Dunks, C.R.T.T., R.C.P.
Robert Tearse, M.D.
503-686-7224/fax: 503-686-3765
E-mail: CDunks@peacehealth.org

Sleep Disorders Center
Rogue Valley Medical Center
2825 East Barnett Road
Medford, OR 97504
Eric Overland, M.D.
Michael Schwartz, R.P.S.G.T.
Nic Butkov, R.P.S.G.T.
541-608-4320/fax: 541-608-5890

**Legacy Good Samaritan Sleep
Disorders Center**
Neurology, T-302
1015 Northwest Twenty-second
Avenue
Portland, OR 97210
John J. Greve, M.D., Medical Director
Jan White, Manager
503-413-7540/fax: 503-413-6919

Pacific Sleep Program
1849 Northwest Kearney, Suite 202
Portland, OR 97209
Gerald B. Rich, M.D.
503-228-4414/fax: 503-228-7293

E-mail: Sleep@snoreweb.com
Web site: www.snoreweb.com

Sleep Disorders Center
Providence St. Vincent Medical
Center
9205 Southwest Barnes Road
Portland, OR 97225
Lyn Miskowicz, Coordinator
Keith Hyde
503-216-2010/fax: 503-216-2614
E-mail: lmiskowicz@providence.org

**Salem Hospital Sleep Disorders
Center**
Salem Hospital
665 Winter Street, SE
Salem, OR 97309-5014
Mark T. Gabr, M.D.
*Stephen J. Baughman, R.R.T.,
R.P.S.G.T.*
503-370-5170/fax: 503-375-4722
E-mail: SJBaug@SalemHospital.org

MCMC Sleep Studies Lab*
Mid-Columbia Medical Center
1700 East 19th
The Dalles, OR 97058
Michael Wacker
541-296-7724/fax: 541-296-7606

PENNSYLVANIA

Sleep Disorders Center
Abington Memorial Hospital
1200 Old York Road
Rorer Building, 2nd Floor
Abington, PA 19001
B. Franklin Diamond, M.D.
Albert D. Wagman, M.D.
Kevin R. Booth, M.D.
215-481-2226/fax: 215-481-2730
E-mail: BFD13042@home.com
Web site: www.amh.org

Sacred Heart Sleep Disorders Center
Sacred Heart Hospital
421 Chew Street
Allentown, PA 18102-3490
William R. Pistone, D.O.
Ross Futerfas, M.D.
K. Alexander Haraldsted, M.D.
David J. Brooks, R.R.T., R.P.S.G.T.
610-776-5333/fax: 610-776-5110
E-mail: shh_sleep@juno.com

Sleep Disorders Center
Lower Bucks Hospital
501 Bath Road
Bristol, PA 19007
Howard J. Lee, M.D.
215-785-9752/fax: 215-785-9068

Penn Center for Sleep Disorders
800 West State Street
Doylestown, PA 18901
Richard J. Schwab, M.D.
Allan I. Pack, M.D., Ph.D.
Louis Metzger
215-345-5003/fax: 215-345-5047

Sleep Disorders Center of Lancaster
Lancaster General Hospital
555 North Duke Street
Lancaster, PA 17604-3555

Harshadkumar B. Patel, M.D.
James M. O'Connor, R.P.S.G.T.,
M.P.A.
717-290-5910/fax: 717-290-4964

Saint Mary Sleep/Wake Disorder Center
Langhorne-Newtown Road
Langhorne, PA 19047
Howard J. Lee, M.D., Medical Director
James J. Burke, Administrative Director
215-741-6744/fax: 215-741-6695

Sleep Medicine Services
Paoli Memorial Hospital
255 West Lancaster Avenue
Paoli, PA 19301
Mark R. Pressman, Ph.D.
Donald D. Peterson, M.D.
610-645-3400/fax: 610-645-2291
E-mail: pressmanm@mlhs.org

Center for Sleep Medicine
Department of Neurology
MCP—Hahnemann University
3200 Henry Avenue
Philadelphia, PA 19129
June M. Fry, M.D., Ph.D., Director
215-842-4250/fax: 215-848-3850

Penn Center for Sleep Disorders
University of Pennsylvania Medical Center
3400 Spruce Street, 11 Gates West
Philadelphia, PA 19104
Allan I. Pack, M.D., Ph.D.
Richard J. Schwab, M.D.

Louis F. Metzger
215-662-7772/fax: 215-349-8038
E-mail:
loumetzg@mail.med.upenn.edu

Pennsylvania Hospital Sleep Disorders Center
Pennsylvania Hospital
Eighth and Spruce Streets
Philadelphia, PA 19107
Charles R. Cantor, M.D.
Ronald L. Kotler, M.D.
215-829-7079/fax: 215-829-5630

Sleep Disorders Center
Thomas Jefferson University
1015 Walnut Street, Suite 319
Philadelphia, PA 19107
Karl Doghramji, M.D.
215-955-6175/fax: 215-955-9783
E-mail: karl.doghramji@mail.tju.edu

Temple Sleep Disorders Center
Temple University Hospital
3401 North Broad Street
Rock Pavilion, 4th Floor
Philadelphia, PA 19140
Samuel Krachman, D.O.
Grace R. Denault, B.A., R.P.S.G.T.
215-707-8163/fax: 215-707-3876
E-mail: DenaulGr@tuhsmsl.tuhi.
temple.edu

University Services
6561 Roosevelt Boulevard
Philadelphia, PA 19149
Irvin M. Gerson, M.D.
Benjamin Gerson, M.D.
215-535-3335/fax: 215-743-7786
E-mail: mmisero@chesco.com
Web site: www.uservices.com

Pulmonary Sleep Evaluation Laboratory*
University of Pittsburgh Medical Center
Montefiore University Hospital
3459 Fifth Avenue, S639
Pittsburgh, PA 15213
Nancy Kern, C.R.T.T., R.P.S.G.T.
Mark H. Sanders, M.D.
Patrick J. Strollo, M.D.
412-692-2880/fax: 412-692-2888

Sleep and Chronobiology Center
Western Psychiatric Institute and Clinic
3811 O'Hara Street
Pittsburgh, PA 15213-2593
Charles F. Reynolds III, M.D.
412-624-2246/fax: 412-624-2841

University Services
1133 High Street
Pottstown, PA 19464
Irvin M. Gerson, M.D.
Benjamin Gerson, M.D.
610-326-6737/fax: 610-326-7751
E-mail: mmisero@chesco.com
Web site: www.uservices.com

Crozer Sleep Disorders Center at Taylor Hospital
175 East Chester Pike
Ridley Park, PA 19078
Calvin Stafford, M.D., Clinical Director
610-595-6272/fax: 610-595-6273
E-mail: staffordt@dvol.com

Sleep Disorders Center
Community Medical Center
1822 Mulberry Street
Scranton, PA 18510
S. Ramakrishna, M.D., F.C.C.P.
717-969-8931

Sleep Disorders Center
Mercy Hospital
25 Church Street
Wilkes-Barre, PA 18765

John Della Rosa, M.D.
570-826-3410/fax: 570-820-6658

Sleep Medicine Services
Lankenau Hospital
100 Lancaster Avenue
Wynnewood, PA 19096
Mark R. Pressman, Ph.D.
Donald D. Peterson, M.D.
610-645-3400/fax: 610-642-2291
E-mail: pressmanm@MLHS.org

RHODE ISLAND
No Accredited Member Centers

SOUTH CAROLINA

Roper Sleep/Wake Disorders Center
Roper Hospital
316 Calhoun Street
Charleston, SC 29401-1125
William T. Dawson, Jr., M.D.
Wayne C. Vial, M.D.
Graham C. Scott, M.D.
John A. Mitchell, M.D.
Tim Fultz, M.S., R.R.T., R.P.S.G.T.
843-724-2246/fax: 843-724-2765
E-mail: tim.fultz@carealliance.com
Web site:
   www.carealliance.com/sleeplab/
   default.html

**Sleep Disorders Center of South
   Carolina**
Baptist Medical Center
Taylor at Marion Street
Columbia, SC 29220
Richard Bogan, M.D., F.C.C.P.
Sharon S. Ellis, M.D., Neonatologist
803-296-5847 or 800-368-1971/
   fax: 803-296-3080
Web site: www.sleep-sdca.com

**Southeast Regional Sleep Disorders
   Center Easley**
200 Fleetwood Drive, P.O. Box 2129
Easley, SC 29640
*Freddie E. Wilson, M.D., Medical
   Director*
Katrinka Scalise
864-855-7200/fax: 864-627-9301

Sleep Disorders Center
Greenville Memorial Hospital
701 Grove Road
Greenville, SC 29605
Don McMahan
864-455-8916/fax: 864-455-4670

**Southeast Regional Sleep Disorders
   Center**
440A Roper Mountain Road
Greenville, SC 29615
*Freddie E. Wilson, M.D., Medical
   Director*

Cathy DeJong, R.R.T., R.P.S.G.T.,
  R.C.P., Clinical Manager
Katrinka Scalise, Facility Manager
864-627-5337/fax: 864-627-9301

Carolinas Sleep Services
1665 Herlong Court, Suite B
Rock Hill, SC 29732
Michael A. Stolzenbach, R.P.S.G.T.,
  Manager
William C. Sherrill, M.D., Medical
  Director
803-817-1915

Sleep Disorders Center
Spartanburg Regional Medical
  Center
101 East Wood Street
Spartanburg, SC 29303
Shari Angel Newman, R.P.S.G.T.
864-560-6904/fax: 864-560-7083
E-mail: snewman@srhs.com

SOUTH DAKOTA

Sleep Center
Rapid City Regional Hospital
353 Fairmont Boulevard
P.O. Box 6000
Rapid City, SD 57709
K. Alan Kelts, M.D., Ph.D.
Terry Anderson, B.S., R.R.C.P.
605-341-8037/fax: 605-341-1924

Sleep Disorders Center
Sioux Valley Hospital
1100 South Euclid
Sioux Falls, SD 57117-5039
Liz Grav
605-333-6302/fax: 605-333-4402
E-mail: gravl@siouxvalley.org

TENNESSEE

Summit Center for Sleep Related
  Breathing Disorders*
Summit Medical Center
5655 First Boulevard,
  MOB–Suite 401
Hermitage, TN 37076
Timothy L. Morgenthaler, M.D.
Lee Ann Covington, R.R.T.,
  R.P.S.G.T.
615-316-3495/fax: 615-316-3493

Sleep Disorders Laboratory*
Regional Hospital of Jackson
367 Hospital Boulevard
Jackson, TN 38303

Thomas W. Ellis, M.D.
David M. Larsen, M.D.
Charlie Carroll, R.P.S.G.T.
901-661-2148/fax: 901-661-2441

Sleep Disorders Center
Fort Sanders Regional Medical
  Center
1901 West Clinch Avenue
Knoxville, TN 37916
Thomas G. Higgins, M.D.
Bert A. Hampton, M.D.
C. Keith Hulse, Ph.D.
865-541-1375/fax: 865-541-1714

Sleep Disorders Center
St. Mary's Medical Center
900 East Oak Hill Avenue
Knoxville, TN 37917-4556
William Finley, Ph.D., Director
423-545-6746/fax: 423-545-3115
E-mail: bFinley@notes.mercy.com

BMH Sleep Disorders Center
Baptist Memorial Hospital
899 Madison Avenue
Memphis, TN 38146
Robert Schriner, M.D.
Sharon Burt, R.P.S.G.T.
901-227-5337/fax: 901-227-5652
E-mail: robertschriner@bmhcc.org

Sleep Disorders Center
Methodist Hospitals of Memphis
1265 Union Avenue
Memphis, TN 38104
Kristin W. Lester, Manager
Jim Donaldson, Supervisor
Robert Neal Aguillard, M.D., Medical
    Director
Srinath Bellur, M.D., Assistant
    Medical Director
901-726-REST/fax: 901-726-7395

Sleep Disorders Center
Middle Tennessee Medical Center
400 North Highland Avenue
Murfreesboro, TN 37130

Timothy J. Hoelscher, Ph.D.
William H. Noah, M.D.
615-849-4811/fax: 615-849-4833

Baptist Sleep Center
Baptist Hospital
2000 Church Street
Nashville, TN 37236
J. Michael Bolds, M.D., Director
Stephen J. Heyman, M.D., Co-Director
615-329-7806/fax: 615-284-4781

Sleep Disorders Center
Centennial Medical Center
2300 Patterson Street
Nashville, TN 37203
David A. Jarvis, M.D.
Marcie T. Poe, R.P.S.G.T.
615-342-1670/fax: 615-342-1655

Sleep Disorders Center
Saint Thomas Hospital
P.O. Box 380
Nashville, TN 37202
J. Brevard Haynes, Jr., M.D.
Susan L. Snyder, Ph.D.
615-222-2068/fax: 615-222-6456

TEXAS

NWTH Sleep Disorders Center
Northwest Texas Hospital
P.O. Box 1110
Amarillo, TX 79175
Michael Westmoreland, M.D.
John Moss, C.R.T.T.
806-354-1954/fax: 806-351-4293

Sleep Disorders Center for Children
Children's Medical Center of Dallas
1935 Motor Street
Dallas, TX 75235
Roya Tompkins
John Herman, Ph.D.
Joel Steinberg, M.D.

214-456-2793/fax: 214-456-8740
E-mail:
    joherma@childmed.dallas.tx.us

Sleep Medicine Institute
Presbyterian Hospital of Dallas
8200 Walnut Hill Lane
Dallas, TX 75231
Philip M. Becker, M.D.
Andrew O. Jamieson, M.D.
Wolfgang Schmidt-Nowara, M.D.
214-345-8563/fax: 214-750-4621
E-mail: SMAT@sleepmed.com
Web site: www.sleepmed.com

Sleep Disorders Center
Columbia Medical Center East
10301 Gateway West
El Paso, TX 79925
Gonzalo Diaz, M.D.
Jean R. Joseph-Vanderpool, M.D.
Elizabeth Baird, R.P.S.G.T.
915-594-5882/fax: 915-595-9641

Sleep Disorders Center
Providence Memorial Hospital
2001 North Oregon
El Paso, TX 79902
Gonzalo Diaz, M.D., F.C.C.P.
Joseph Arteaga, R.P.S.G.T.
915-577-6152/fax: 915-577-6119

Sleep Consultants, Inc.
1521 Cooper Street
Fort Worth, TX 76104
Edgar Lucas, Ph.D.
C. Marshall Bradshaw, M.D.
John R. Burk, M.D.
Kristyna M. Hartse, Ph.D.
817-332-7433/fax: 817-336-2159
E-mail: info@sleepconsultants.com
Web site: www.sleepconsultants.com

Sleep Center
Spring Branch Medical Center
8850 Long Point Road
Houston, TX 77055
Todd J. Swick, M.D.
713-984-3519/fax: 713-722-3248
E-mail: tswick@ix.metcom.com

Sleep Disorders Center
Department of Psychiatry
Baylor College of Medicine and VA
    Medical Center
One Baylor Plaza
Houston, TX 77030
Constance Moore, M.D., Director
Max Hirshkowitz, Ph.D., Co-Director
713-798-4886 or 713-794-7563/fax:
    713-798-4099 or 713-794-7558
E-mail: maxh@bcm.tmc.edu or
    cmoore@bcm.tmc.edu

Sleep Disorders Center
Hermann Hospital
6411 Fannin Street
Houston, TX 77030
Richard Castriotta, M.D.
713-704-2337/fax: 713-704-5586
E-mail:
    rcastrio@heart.meduth.tmc.edu
Web site:
    www.salu.net/hermannsleep/

Sleep Disorders Center
Scott and White Clinic
2401 South 31st Street
Temple, TX 76508
Francisco Perez-Guerra, M.D.
254-724-2554/fax: 254-724-2497
E-mail: fperez-guerra@mailbox.
    sw.org

UTAH

Intermountain Sleep Disorders Center of Murray Cottonwood Hospital
5770 South, 300 East
Murray, UT 84106
James M. Walker, Ph.D.
Robert J. Farney, M.D.
801-269-2015/fax: 801-269-2948

Intermountain Sleep Disorders Center
LDS Hospital
Eighth Avenue and C Street
Salt Lake City, UT 84143
James M. Walker, Ph.D.
Robert J. Farney, M.D.

801-321-3617/fax: 801-321-5110
E-mail: ldjwalke@ihc.com

Sleep Disorders Center
University of Utah Hospitals and Clinic
50 North Medical Drive
Salt Lake City, UT 84132
Christopher R. Jones, M.D., Ph.D., Co-Medical Director
.Kenneth R. Casey, M.D., F.C.C.P., Co-Medical Director
Laura Czajkowski, Ph.D.
Linda Webster, R.E.E.G./E.P.T., R.P.S.G.T., Manager
801-581-2016/fax: 801-585-3249

VERMONT
No Accredited Member Centers

VIRGINIA

Fairfax Sleep Disorders Center
3289 Woodburn Road, Suite 360
Annandale, VA 22003
Konrad W. Bakker, M.D.
Marc Raphaelson, M.D.
703-876-9870

Virginia-Carolina Sleep Disorders Center
159 Executive Drive, Suite D
Danville, VA 24541
Jacalyn A. Nelson, M.D., Medical Director
Della C. Williams, M.D.
Mugabala B. Aswath, M.D.
William Underwood, R.P.S.G.T.
Nancy Craig Williams, B.S., R.P.S.G.T.

804-792-2209/fax: 804-799-8037
E-mail: vanc.sleep@juno.com

Sleep Disorders Center for Adults and Children
Eastern Virginia Medical School
Sentara Norfolk General Hospital
600 Gresham Drive
Norfolk, VA 23507
J. Catesby Ware, Ph.D.
Jeffery A. Scott, M.D.
Nancy Fishback, M.D.
A. J. Quaranta, M.D.
Robert D. Vorona, M.D.
757-668-3322/fax: 757-668-2628
E-mail: sleep@evms.edu
Web site: www.evms.edu/sleep/

Sleep Disorders Center
Medical College of Virginia
2529 Professional Road
Richmond, VA 23235
Rakesh K. Sood, M.D.
804-323-2255/fax: 804-323-2262

Sleep Disorders Center of Virginia
1800 Glenside Drive, Suite 103
Richmond, VA 23226
Read F. McGehee, Jr., M.D.
804-285-0100/fax: 804-285-2458
E-mail: sleepva@i2020.net

Sleep Disorders Center
Carilion Roanoke Community
    Hospital
P.O. Box 12946
Roanoke, VA 24029
William S. Elias, M.D.
540-985-8526/fax: 540-985-4963

Sleep Disorders Center
Obici Hospital
1900 North Main Street
P.O. Box 1100

Suffolk, VA 23439-1100
Frances Davidson, R.T.,
    Administrative Director
Leah S. Pixley, C.R.T., R.E.E.G.T.,
    R.P.S.G.T., Clinical Manager
Hemang Shah, M.D., Medical Director
757-934-4450/fax: 757-934-4278
E-mail: lpixley@obici.com
Web site: www.obici.com

Sleep Disorders Center
Virginia Beach General Hospital
1060 First Colonial Road
Virginia Beach, VA 23454
Bruce Johnson, M.D.
Yvonne Wright-Dunn, B.A.,
    R.P.S.G.T.
757-395-8168/fax: 757-395-6337
E-mail: ywright-dunn@tidehealth.
    com

WASHINGTON

ARMC Sleep Apnea Laboratory*
Auburn Regional Medical Center,
    Plaza One
202 North Division
Auburn, WA 98001
Julie Holdaas, R.P.S.G.T.
Leslie Cuiper, M.D., Medical Director
253-804-2809/fax: 253-735-7599

**St. Clare Sleep Related Breathing
    Disorders Clinic***
St. Clare Hospital
11315 Bridgeport Way, SW
Lakewood, WA 98499

Arthur Knodel, M.D.
Erin Salsbury, R.P.S.G.T.
253-581-6951/fax: 253-512-2793

**Sleep Disorders Center for
    Southwest Washington**
Providence St. Peter Hospital
413 North Lilly Road
Olympia, WA 98506
Kim A. Chase, R.P.S.G.T.
John L. Brottem, M.D.
360-493-7436/fax: 360-493-4173

Sleep Center at Valley
Valley Medical Center
400 South Forty-third Street
Renton, WA 98055
Carla J. Hellekson, M.D., F.A.P.A.
William J. DePaso, M.D., F.C.C.P.
425-656-5340/fax: 425-656-5436
E-mail: Barry_Stone@Valleymed.org
Web site: www.valleymed.org

Columbia Sleep Lab*
780 Swift Boulevard, Suite 130
Richland, WA 99352
W. S. Klipper, M.D., F.A.C.C.P.
Claudia Havner, C.R.T.T., N.R.T.,
P.S.G.T.
509-943-6166/fax: 509-943-8621
E-mail: Sleepy2400@hotmail.com

Richland Sleep Disorders Center
800 Swift Boulevard, Suite 260
Richland, WA 99352
A. Pat Hamner, Jr., M.D.
509-946-4632/fax: 509-942-0118
E-mail: phamner@owt.com
Web site: www.richsleep.com

Highline Sleep Disorder Center
Highline Community Hospital
14212 Ambaum Boulevard, SW,
 Suite 201
Seattle, WA 98166
Margaret Moen, M.D., Medical
Director
John Lovelace, R.R.T.
Lamont Porter, R.C.P.
206-325-7396/fax: 206-242-2562

Providence Sleep Disorders Center
500 17th Avenue, Department 4W
Seattle, WA 98122
Ralph A. Pascualy, M.D.
Sarah E. Stolz, M.D.

206-320-2575/fax: 206-320-3339
E-mail: lpascualy@aol.com
Web site: www.sleep.org

Seattle Sleep Disorders Center
Swedish Medical Center/Ballard
P.O. Box 70707
Seattle, WA 98107-1507
Gary A. DeAndrea, M.D.
Noel T. Johnson, D.O.
Richard P. Swanson, R.P.S.G.T.,
C.R.T.T.
206-781-6359/fax: 206-781-6196
E-mail:
 rick.swanson@mail.swedish.org
Web site: www.swedish.org

Virginia Mason Medical Center
 Sleep Disorders Center
Virginia Mason Hospital, H10-SDC
925 Seneca Street
Seattle, WA 98101-2742
Neely E. Pardee, M.D.
Kenneth R. Casey, M.D.
Steven H. Kirtland, M.D.
Nigel J. Ball, D.Phil.
206-625-7180/fax: 206-341-0447
E-mail: sdcsdc@vmmc.org

Sleep Disorders Center
Sacred Heart Doctors Building
105 West Eighth Avenue, Suite 418
Spokane, WA 99204
Elizabeth Hurd, R.P.S.G.T.
Jeffrey C. Elmer, M.D.
509-455-4895/fax: 509-626-4578
E-mail: HURDE@SHMC.ORG

Kathryn Severyns Dement Sleep
 Disorders Center
St. Mary Medical Center
401 West Poplar, P.O. Box 1047
Walla Walla, WA 99362

Richard D. Simon, Jr., M.D.
Kevin Hurlburt, R.P.S.G.T.
509-522-5845/fax: 509-522-5744
E-mail: sleepcenter@smmc.com
Web site: www.smmc.com/sleep

WEST VIRGINIA

Sleep Disorders Center
Charleston Area Medical Center
501 Morris Street, P.O. Box 1393
Charleston, WV 25325
George Zaldivar, M.D., F.C.C.P.
Karen Stewart, R.R.T., Manager
304-348-7507/fax: 304-348-3373

St. Mary's Regional Sleep Center
St. Mary's Hospital
2400 First Avenue
Huntington, WV 25702
William R. Beam, M.D., F.C.C.P.

David Imhoff, R.R.T., R.N., M.B.A.
Kathy Johnson, R.E.E.G./E.P.T.,
R.P.S.G.T.
304-526-1881/fax: 304-526-1886
E-mail: dimhoff@ezwv.com

PM Sleep Medicine
3803 Emerson Avenue
P.O. Box 4179
Parkersburg, WV 26104
Michael A. Morehead, M.D.
M. Barry Louden, M.D.
304-485-5041/fax: 304-485-5678

WISCONSIN

Sleep Disorders Center
Appleton Medical Center
1818 North Meade Street
Appleton, WI 54911
Kevin C. Garrett, M.D.
920-738-6460/fax: 920-831-5000

**Marshfield Clinic Sleep Disorders
Center**
Chippewa Center Sleep Laboratory
2655 County Highway 1
Chippewa Falls, WI 54729
Mary Jacks, R.P.S.G.T., R.E.E.G.T.
Nancy Bender Hausman, M.D.
715-726-4136/fax: 715-726-4173
E-mail: Hausmann@mfldclin.edu

**Luther/Midelfort Sleep Disorders
Center**
Luther Hospital/Midelfort Clinic
Mayo Health System
1221 Whipple Street, P.O. Box 4105
Eau Claire, WI 54702-4105
Donn Dexter, M.D.
David Nye, M.D.
715-838-3165/fax: 715-838-3845
E-mail: dexter.donn@mayo.edu

**St. Vincent Hospital Sleep Disorders
Center**
St. Vincent Hospital
P.O. Box 13508
Green Bay, WI 54307-3508
John Andrews, M.D.

John Stevenson, M.D.
Paula Van Ert, R.P.S.G.T.
920-431-3041/fax: 920-433-8010
E-mail: pvanert@svgb.org

Sleep Disorders Laboratory*
Bellin Hospital
744 South Webster Avenue
Green Bay, WI 54301
John Stevenson, M.D.
Lee Kvaley, R.R.T.
920-433-7451/fax: 920-433-7453
E-mail: slplab@bellin.org

Wisconsin Sleep Disorders Center
Gundersen Lutheran
1836 South Avenue
La Crosse, WI 54601
Alan D. Pratt, M.D.
608-782-7300 Ext. 2870/
    fax: 608-791-4466
E-mail: AlanPratt/Pulm/
    lax/gundluth@gundluth.org

**Comprehensive Sleep Disorders
    Center**
D6/662 Clinical Science Center
University of Wisconsin Hospitals
    and Clinics
600 Highland Avenue
Madison, WI 53792
Steven M. Weber, Ph.D.
John C. Jones, M.D.
608-263-2387/fax: 608-263-0412
E-mail: smweber2@facstaff.wisc.edu
    or jones@neurology.wisc.edu

Sleep Disorders Center
St. Marys Hospital Medical Center
707 South Mills Street
Madison, WI 53715
Steve Dalebroux
Kathryn L. Middleton, M.D.
608-258-5266/fax: 608-258-6176

**Sleep Disorders Center Meriter
    Hospital**
Meriter Hospital, Inc.
202 South Park Street
Madison, WI 53715
Lyman Riley, Manager
Mary Klink, M.D., Medical Director
608-267-5938/fax: 608-267-6540
E-mail: lriley@meriter.com

Marshfield Sleep Disorders Center
Marshfield Clinic
1000 North Oak Avenue
Marshfield, WI 54449
Jody Scherr, R.P.S.G.T., R.E.E.G.T.
Kevin Ruggles, M.D.
715-387-5397/fax: 715-387-5240
E-mail: Rugglesk@mfldclin.edu

**Milwaukee Regional Sleep Disorders
    Center**
Columbia Hospital
2025 East Newport Avenue,
    Suite 426Y
Milwaukee, WI 53211
Marvin Wooten, M.D.
Joni Tombari, Program Director
414-961-4650/fax: 414-961-4545

St. Luke's Sleep Disorders Center
St. Luke's Medical Center
2801 West Kinnickinnic River
    Parkway, Suite 445
Milwaukee, WI 53215
David Arnold, R.P.S.G.T.

Michael N. Katzoff, M.D.
414-649-5288/fax: 414-649-5875
E-mail: dave_arnold@aurora.org or
  mnka@aol.com

WYOMING
No Accredited Member Centers

Notes

Chapter 1. How and Why We Sleep

Asplund, R., and H. Aberg. Nocturnal micturation, sleep, and well-being in women of ages 40–64 years. *Maturitas* 1996; 24 (102):73–81.

Carskadon, M. A. Patterns of sleep and sleepiness in adolescents. *Pediatrician* 1990; 17:5–12.

Coren, S. The prevalence of self-reported sleep disturbance in young adults. *Int. J. Neurosci.*1004; 79(1–2):67–73.

Ehlers, C. L., and D. I. Kupfer. Slow-wave sleep: Do young adult men and women age differently? *J. Sleep Res.* 1997; 6:211–15.

Gallup Organization. Sleep in America: A National Survey of U.S. Adults. National Sleep Foundation, 1991.

———.Sleep in America: A National Survey of U.S. Adults. National Sleep Foundation, 1995.

Hall, M., et al. Sleep as a mediator of the stress-immune relationship. *Psychosomatic Med.* 1998; 60:48–51.

Hughes, R. J. , R. L. Sack, and A. J. Lewy. The role of melatonin and circadian phase in age-related sleep-maintenance insomnia: assessment in a clinical trial of melatonin replacement. *Sleep* 1998; 21(1):52–68.

Louis Harris & Associates. *Sleepiness, Pain and the Workplace.* National Sleep Foundation, 1997.

Johns, M. W. A new model for measuring daytime sleepiness: The Epworth Sleepiness Scale. *Sleep* 1991; 14:540.

Jouvet, M. Recherches sur les structures nerveuses et les mécanismes responsables des differentes phases du sommeil physiologique. *Arch. Ital. Biol.* 1962; 100:125.

Manber, R., et al. The effects of regularizing sleep-wake schedules on daytime sleepiness. *Sleep* 1996; 19(5):432–41.

McCartt, A., chairman, New York State Taskforce on the Impact of Drowsy Driving. Institute for Traffic Safety Management and Research, Albany, New York, December 1994.

Mitler, E. A., and M. M. Mitler. *101 Questions About Sleep and Dreams,* 5th ed. Del Mar, CA: Wakefulness Sleep Education and Research Foundation, 1995.

Mitler, M. M., D. R. Kripke, and M. R. Klauber. No relationship between amount of sleep and amount of exercise. *Sleep Research* 1999; H399.I.

Morin, C. M., D. Gibson, and J. Wade. Self-reported sleep and mood disturbance in chronic pain patients. *Clinical J. Pain* 1998; 14:311–14.

Phillips, B. A., and F. J. Danner. Cigarette smoking and sleep disturbance. *Arch. Intern. Med.* 1995; 155(7):734–37.

Rediker, N. S., et al. Sleep patterns in women after coronary artery bypass surgery. *Appl. Nurs. Res.* 1996; 9(3):115–22.

Roehrs, T., D. Beare, F. Zorick, and T. Roth. Sleepiness and ethanol effects of simulated driving. *Alcohol Clin. Exp. Res.* 1994; 18(1):154–58.

Roth, T., et al. Comparative "dose" effect of ethanol and sleep loss. *Sleep Research* 1999; H150.I.

Todd Arnedt, J., and A. W. MacLean. Simulated driving performance during sleep loss and following alcohol consumption: independent versus combined effects. *Sleep Research* 1999; H403.I.

Umlauf, M., and E. Kurtzer, et al. Sleep-disordered breathing as a mechanism for nocturia: preliminary findings. *Ostomy/Wound Management,* December 1999; vol. 45; no. 12:52–60.

Vgontzas, A. N., et al. Circadian interleukin-6 secretion and quantity and depth of sleep. *Endocrinol. Metab.* 1999; 84:2603–7.

Wauquier, A. Aging and changes in phasic events during sleep. *Physiol. Behav.* 1993; 54(4):803–6.

Williams, R. L., J. Karacan, and C. J. Hursch. *Electroencephalography of Human Sleep: Clinical Applications.* New York: Wiley, 1974.

Chapter 2. Our Raging Hormones

Altura, B., et al., Premenstrual syndrome. *Fertil. and Steril.* 1998; 69; 958–62.

Baker, A., S. Simpson, and D. Dawson. Sleep disruption and mood changes associated with menopause. *J. Psychomsom. Res.* 1997; 43(4):359–69.

The Complete German Commission E. Monographs: Therapeutic Guide to Herbal Medicines. American Botanical Council, 1998.

Czeizler, C., et al. Melatonin levels do not fall with age. *Am. J. Med.* 1999; 107: 422–36.

Driver, H. S., et al. Sleep and the sleep electroencephalogram across the menstrual cycle in young healthy women. *J. Clin. Endocrinol. Metab.* 1996; 81(2):728–35.

Driver, H. S., and F. C. Baker, Menstrual factors in sleep. *Sleep Med. Rev.* 1998; 213–29. Taken from paper on menstruation-related periodic hypersomnia: a case study with successful treatment. *Neurology* 1982; 32:1376–79.

Erlik, Y., et al. Association of waking episodes with menopausal hot flashes. *JAMA* 1981; 245:1741–44.

Fast, A., et al. Night backache in pregnancy: Hypothetical pathophysico-psychological mechanisms. *Am. J. Phys. Med. Rehab.* 1989; 69:227–29, cited in Mary V. Seeman, ed., *Gender and Psychopathology.* American Psychiatric Press, 1995.

Feinsilver, S. H., and G. Hertz. Respiration during sleep in pregnancy. *Clin. Chest Med.* 1992; 13:637–46.

Krystal, A. D., J. Edinger, et al. Sleep in perimenopausal and post-menopausal women. *Sleep Med. Rev.* 1998; 2(4):243–53.

Kuh, D. L., M. Wadsworth, and R. Hardy. Women's health in midlife: the influence of the menopausal, social factors and health in earlier life. *Br. J. Obstet. Gynaecol.* 1997; 104(8):923–33. From questionnaire of British women at age 47 with and without natural menopause.

Lee, K. A. Alterations in sleep during pregnancy and postpartum: A review of thirty years of research. *Sleep Med. Rev.* 1998; 2(4):231–42.

Lee, K. A., and D. L. Taylor. Is there a generic midlife woman? The health and symptom experience of employed midlife women, *Journal of the North American Menopause Society* 1996; vol. 3; 3:154–64.

Lee, K. A., M. E. Zaffke, and G. McEnany. Parity and sleep patterns during and after pregnancy. *Obstetrics and Gynecology* 2000; 95(1):14–18.

Lee, K. A., M. E. Zaffke, G. McEnany, and K. Hoehler. Sleep and fatigue before, during and after pregnancy. *Sleep Res.* 1994; 23:416.

Leibenluft, E., P. Fiero, and D. R. Rubinow. Effects of the menstrual cycle on dependent variables in mood disorder research. *Arch. Gen. Psychiat.* 1994; 51:761–81.

Livrea, P., F. M. Puca, A. Barnaba, and L. DiReda. Abnormal central monoamine metabolism in humans with true hypersomnia and sub-wakefulness. *Eur. Neurol.* 1977; 15:71–76.

Manber, R., and R. R. Bootzin. Sleep and the menstrual cycle. *Health Psychol.* 1997; 16(3):209–14.

Manber, R., and R. Armitage. Sex, steroids and sleep: A Review. *Sleep,* 1999; 22(5):540–55.

Menstruation-related periodic hypersomnia: a case study with successful treatment. *Neurology* 1982; 32:1376–79.

Miller, J. "Beyond the Blues: Postpartum Reactivity and the Biology of Attachment." Presentation to American Psychiatric Association Annual Meeting, 1996, and Interview, quoted in R. Baron-Faust, *Mental Wellness for Women.* New York: Morrow, 1997.

Murphy, P., and S. Campbell. Luteinizing hormone and sleep in post-menopausal women. *Sleep* 1999; 21(Suppl):300.

Polo-Kantola, P., et al. When does estrogen replacement therapy improve sleep quality? *Am. J. Obstet. Gynecol.* 1998; 178(5):1002–9.

Purdie, D. W., et al. Hormone replacement therapy, sleep quality, and psychological well-being. *Br. J. Obstet. Gynaecol.* 1995; 102(9):735–39.

Reichman, J. *I'm Too Young to Get Old.* New York: Times Books, 1997.

Robins, L. N., and D. A. Regier. *Psychiatric Disorders in America: The Epidemiologic Catchment Area Study.* New York: Free Press, 1991.

Sakahee, et al. Meta-analysis of calcium bioavailability: A comparison of calcium citrate with calcium carbonate. *Am. J. Therapeutics,* November 1999.

Schmidt, P., et al. Differential behavioral effects of gonadal steroids in women with and in those without premenstrual syndrome. *New Eng. J. Med.* 1998; 338(4):209–16.

Schoor, S. J., et al. Sleep patterns in pregnancy: A longitudinal study of polysomnography recordings during pregnancy. *J. Perinatol.* 1998; 18(6pt 1):427–30.

Severino, S., and M. Moline. *Premenstrual Syndrome: A Clinician's Guide.* New York: Guilford Press, 1989.

Sharf, M., et al. Effects of estrogen replacement therapy on rates of cyclic alternating patterns and hot-flash events during sleep in postmenopausal women: A pilot study. *Clin. Therap.* 1997; 19(2):304–11.

Spitzer, R., et al. Jet lag: Clinical features, validation of a new syndrome-specific scale and lack of response to melatonin in a randomized, double-blind trial. *Am. J. Psychiat.* September 1999; p. 1392.

Steiger, A., et al. Effects of hormones on sleep. *Hor. Res.* 1998; 49:125–30.

Stone, A., and T. Pearlstein. Evaluation and treatment of changes in mood, sleep and sexual functioning associated with menopause. Primary care of the mature women. *Obstet. Gynecol. Clin. N.A.* 1994; 21(2):391–403.

Swain, A. M., et al. A prospective study of sleep: Mood and cognitive function in postpartum and non-postpartum women. *Obstet. Gynecol.* 1997; 90(3):381–86.

Thys-Jacobs, S. Calcium carbonate and the premenstrual syndrome: Effects on premenstrual and menstrual symptoms. *Am. J. Obstet. Gynecol.* 1998; 179(2):444–52.

Waldstreicher, J., et al. Gender differences in the temporal organization of prolactin PRL secretion: evidence for a sleep-independent circadian rhythm of circulating PRL levels—a clinical research center study. *J. Clin. Endocrinol. Metab.* 1996; 81(4):1483–87.

Woodward, S., and R. R. Freedman. The thermoregulatory effects of menopausal HF on sleep. *Sleep* 1994; 6:497–501.

Wyatt, K. M., et al. Study of vitamin B-6 and premenstrual syndrome. *Br. Med. J.* 1999; 318:1375–81. Announcement by the National Heart, Lung and Blood Institute, April 4, 2000, based on preliminary data from the Women's Health Initiative.

Chapter 3. Women's Ages and Stages of Sleep

Abrams, P., and A. Wein. *The Overactive Bladder: A Widespread and Treatable Condition,* Uppsala, Sweden: Pharmacia & Upjohn, 1998.

Asplund, R., and H. Aberg. Sleep and cardiac symptoms amongst women aged 40–64. *J. Intern. Med.* 1998; 243:209–13.

Bliwise, D. L. Sleep in normal aging and dementia. *Sleep* 1993; 16:40–81.

Buysee, D. J., et al. Patterns of sleep episodes in young and elderly adults in a 36-hour constant routine. *Sleep* 1993; 16(7): 632–37.

Coble, P. A., et al. Childbearing in women with and without a history of affective disorder. II. Electroencephalographic sleep. *Compr. Psych.* 1994; 35(3):215–24.

Coren, S. The prevalence of self-reported sleep disturbances in young adults. *Int. J. Neurosci.* 1994; 79(1–2): 67–73.

Galinsky, E., et al. *National Study of the Changing Work Force.* New York: Families and Work Institute, 1993.

Hughes, R. J., R. L. Sack, and A. J. Lewy. The role of melatonin and circadian phase in age related sleep-maintenance insomnia: Assessment in a clinical trial of melatonin replacement. *Sleep* 1998; 21(1):52–68.

Kobayashi, R., et al. Gender differences in the sleep of middle-aged individuals. *Psych. Clin. Neurosci.* 1998; 52(2):186–87.

Kushi et al. University of Minnesota School of Public Health Study, 1997. Reported in the *New York Times,* April 23, 1997.

Lee, K. A. Alterations in sleep during pregnancy and postpartum: A review of thirty years of research. *Sleep Med. Rev.* 1998; 2(4):231–42.

Lee, K. A., and DeJoseph. Sleep disturbance, vitality and fatigue among a select group of employed childbearing women. *Sleep* 1992; 15(6):493–98.

Lee, K. A., G. McEnany, and D. Weekes. Gender differences in sleep patterns for early adolescents. *J. Adoles. Health.* 1999; 24:16–20.

Lee, K. A., M. E. Zaffke, G. McEnany, and K. Hoehler. Sleep and fatigue before, during and after pregnancy. *Sleep Res.* 1994; 23:416.

Lentz, M., et al. Effects of selective slow-wave sleep disruption on musculoskeletal pain and fatigue in middle-aged women. *J. Rheumatol.* 1999; 26(7):1586–91.

Leonhardt, D. More bosses encourage napping on the job. *New York Times,* October 13, 1999.

Lusardi, P., et al. Effects of insufficient sleep on blood pressive in hypertensive patients. *Am. J. Hypertension,* May 1996.

Lushinton, K., et al. Daytime melatonin administration in elderly good and poor sleepers: effects on core body temperature and sleep latency. *Sleep* 1997; 20(12):1135–44.

Lusskin, S. *Mood Disorders During Pregnancy and the Post-Partum Period.* Hospital Physician Board Review Manual, *Ob. Gyn.* 1999; 5(2):15–23.

Marshall, N. "The Work/Family Interface and Employed Women's Health." Paper presented to American Psychological Association Conference on Women's Health, May 1994.

The Medical Advisor, The Complete Guide to Alternative and Conventional Treatments, Time-Life Books, 1996.

Mooe, T., et al. Sleep disordered breathing in women: Occurrence and association with coronary disease. *Am. J. Med.* 1996; 101(3):251–56. National Sleep Foundation 2000 Omnibus Sleep in America Poll, April 4, 2000.

Redeker, N. S., et al. Sleep patterns in women after coronary artery bypass surgery. *Appl. Nurs. Res.* 1996; 9(3):115–22.

Schectman, K. B., et al. Gender, self-reported depressive symptoms and sleep disturbance among older community-dwelling persons. FICSIT group. Frailty and injuries: Cooperative studies of intervention techniques. *J. Psychosom. Res.* 1997; 43(5):513–27.

Shaver, J. L., *Family Prac. Res. J.* 1993; 13(4):373–84.

Wisner, K., et al. Pharmacological treatment of depression during pregnancy. *JAMA* 1999; 282(13):1264–69.

Zammit, G. K., et al. Quality of life in people with insomnia. *Sleep* 1999; 22, S2:S379–85.

Chapter 4. Women and Sleep Disorders

Birketvedt, G. S., and A. Stunkard. Behavioral and neuroendocrine characteristics of night-eating syndrome. *JAMA* 1999; 282(7):657–63.

Bootzin, R. R., D. Epstein, and J. M. Wood. Stimulus control instructions. In P. Hauri, ed., *Case Studies in Insomnia.* New York: Plenum Publishing, 1991.

Carskadon, M. A., et al. Effects of menopause and nasal occlusion on breathing during sleep. *Am. J. Respir. Crit. Care. Med.* 1997; 155(1):205–10.

Culebras, A., ed. *Clinical Handbook of Sleep Disorders.* Boston: Butterworth-Heinemann, 1996.

Czeisler, C. A., et al. Chronotherapy: Resetting the circadian clocks of patients with delayed sleep phase insomnia. *Sleep* 4:1, 1981.

Dancy, D., et al. "Retrospective Analysis of Sleep Apnea in Menopausal and Pre-Menopausal Women." Presented May 11, 2000, at the 2000 meeting of the American Thoracic Society.

Diagnostic Classification Steering Committee, M. J. Thorpy, ed. *The International Classification of Sleep Disorders Diagnostic and Coding Manual.* Rochester, MN: American Sleep Disorders Association, 1990.

Dinges, D. F., and R. J. Broughton, eds. *Sleep and Alertness: Chronobiological, Behavioral and Medical Aspects of Napping.* New York: Raven, 1989.

Early, C. J., and J. R. Connors. RLS patients have abnormally reduced CSF ferritin compared to both normals and patient controls. *Sleep* 1999; 22,S:156.

Franklin, K., et al. Hypertension and Fetal Growth. *Chest,* January 4, 2000.

Fujita, S., et al. Surgical corrections of anatomic abnormalities in obstructive sleep apnea syndrome: Uvulopapatopharyngoplasty. *Otolaryngol. Head Neck. Surg.* 1981; 89:923.

Giampiero, P., et al. HRT as a first step treatment of insomnia in post-menopausal women. *Eur. Menopause J.* 1997; 4(4):145–46.

Guilleminault, C., J. Hold, and M. M. Mitler. Clinical overview of the sleep apnea syndromes. In C. Guilleminault and W. C. Dement, eds. *Sleep Apnea Syndromes.* New York: Alan R. Liss, 1978.

Guilleminault, C., et al. Upper airway sleep-disordered breathing in women. *Ann. Intern. Med.* 1995; 122(7):493–501.

Hauri, P. J., and S. Linde. *No More Sleepless Nights.* New York: Wiley, 1996.

Hu, et al. Prospective study of snoring and risk of hypertension in women. *Am. J. Epidemiol.* 1999; 150(8):806–16.

Kiely, J. L., and W. T. Mcnicholas. Bed partners assessment of nasal continuous airway pressure therapy in obstructive sleep apnea. *Chest* 1997; 111(5):1261–65.

Kristoff, N. Alien abduction? Science calls it sleep paralysis. *New York Times,* July 6, 1999.

Kryger, M. H., T. Roth, and W. C. Dement, eds. *Principles and Practice of Sleep Medicine,* 2nd ed. Philadelphia: Saunders, 1994.

Leech, et al. A comparison of men and women with occlusive sleep apnea syndrome. *Chest,* 1998; 94:983–88. Cited in M. Seeman, *Gender and Psychopathology.*

Li, K., et al. "Radiofrequency Volumetric Reduction of the Palate: An Extended Follow-up Study." Paper presented to the American Academy of Otolaryngology, Head and Neck Surgery Foundation Annual Meeting, September 26, 1999.

Lin, L., et al. The sleep disorder canine narcolepsy is caused by mutation in the hypocretin (orexin) receptor 2 gene. *Cell* 1999; 98:365–76.

Mahowald, M., and C. H. Schenck. Dissociated state of wakefulness and sleep. *Neurology* 1992; 42:44–52.

Meyers, J., et al. "Sleep Apnea Therapy Enhances Sexual Functioning." Study presented to American College of Chest Physicians Annual Meeting, October 31, 1999.

Millman, R. P., et al. Body fat distribution and sleep apnea severity in women. *Chest* 1995; 107(2):362–66.

Mignot, et al. *Cell* 1999; 98:365–76.

Moldofsky, H. Fibromyalgia, sleep disorder and chronic fatigue syndrome. *Ciba Foundation Symposium* 1993; 173:262–71.

Mooe, T., et al. Sleep-disordered breathing in women: occurrence and association with coronary artery disease. *Am. J. Med.* 1006; 101(3):251–56.

Morin, C., et al. Behavioral and pharmacological therapies for late-life insomnia: A randomized controlled trial. *JAMA* 1999; 281(11):991–99.

Nieto, F., T. Young et al. Association of sleep-disordered breathing, sleep apnea, and hypertension in a large community-based study. *JAMA* 2000; 283(4):1829–36.

Nishino, S., et al. Underexpression of hypocretin 1 in narcolepsy. *Lancet* 2000; 355:39–40.

Ohayon, M., et al. Sleep paralysis. *Neurology*, April 12, 1999.

Peppard, P., T. Young et al. Prospective study of the association between sleep-disordered breathing and hypertension. *New Engl. J. Med.* 2000; 342(19):1378–84.

Pickett, C. K., et al. Progestin and estrogen reduce sleep-disordered breathing in postmenopausal women. *J. Appl. Physiol.* 1989; 66(4):1656–61.

Powell, N., et al. "A Comparative Model: Reaction Time Performance in Sleep Disordered Breathing Versus Alcohol-Impaired Controls." Study presented to the American Academy of Otolaryngology, Head and Neck Surgery Annual Meeting, September 26, 1999.

Schenk, C. H., and M. W. Mahowald. Review of nocturnal sleep-related eating disorders. *Int. J. Eating Dis.* 1994; 15(4):343–56.

Shaver, J., and L. Landish. *Res. Nursing Health* 1997; 20(3):247–57.

Skaer, T., et al. Psychiatric comorbidity and pharmacological treatment patterns among patients with insomnia. *Clin. Drug. Invest.* 1999; 18(2):161–67.

Spielman, A. J., P. Saskin, and M. J. Thorpy. Treatment of chronic insomnia by restriction of time in bed. *Sleep* 1987; 10:45–56.

Sullivan, C. E., et al. Reversal of obstructive sleep apnea by continuous positive airway pressure applied through the nares. *Lancet* 1981; 1:862.

Valencia-Flores, M., et al. Gender differences in sleep architecture in sleep apnea syndrome. *J. Sleep Res.* 1992; 1:51–53. Cited in Seeman, *Gender and Psychopathology.*

Yaeger, J. Nocturnal eating syndromes: To sleep, perchance to eat. *JAMA*, August 18, 1999; 689–92.

Young, T., et al. The gender bias in sleep apnea diagnosis. *Arch. Intern. Med.* 1996; 156:2445–51.

Young, T. B., et al. The occurrence of sleep-disordered breathing among middle-aged adults. *N. Eng. J. Med.* 1993; 328.

Wilson, K., et al. Overweight males are loudest snorers. *Chest*, March 1999.

Winkleman, J. W. Clinical and polysomnographic features of sleep-related eating disorder. *J. Clin. Psych.* 1998; 59:14–19.

Wirz-Justice, et al. Sleep latency and inadequate vasodilation. *Nature* 1999; 401:36–37.

Zarcone, V. P. Sleep and alcoholism. In M. Chase and E. D. Weitzman, eds., *Sleep Disorders: Basic and Clinical Research. Advances in Sleep Research.* New York: Spectrum, 1983.

Chapter 5. In Your Dreams

Cartwright, R., et al. Role of REM sleep and dream in overnight mood regulation: A study of normal volunteers. *Psych. Res.* 1998; 81:1–8.

Crick, F., and G. R. Mitchinson. The function of dream sleep. *Nature* 1983; 304:111–14.

Dement, W. C., and N. Kleitman. Cyclic variations in EEG during sleep and their relation to eye movements, body motility and dreaming. *Electroencephalogr. Clin. Neurophysiol.* 1957; 9:673.

Freud, S. *The Interpretation of Dreams.*

Gilyatt, P. Sleep may play bigger role in learning and memory. *Harvard Medical School Focus,* March 19, 1999.

Goodson, L. *The Dreams of Women.* New York: Berkley Books, 1995.

Hobson, J. A., and R. W. McCarley. The brain as a dream state generator: An activation-synthesis hypothesis of the dream process. *Am. J. Psych.* 1977; 134:1335.

Kalb, C. What dreams are made of. *Newsweek,* November 8, 1999, p. 77.

Massicotte Pass, C. Sleep dreams of women in the childbearing years: A review of research. *Holistic Nursing Prac.* 1996; 10(4):12–19.

Chapter 6. Sleep and Sex

Baron-Faust, R. *Mental Wellness for Women.* New York: Morrow, 1997.

Boland, B. D., and D. A. Dewsbury. Characteristics of sleep following sexual activity and wheel running in male rats. *Physiol. Behav.* 1971; 6:145–49.

Brissette, S., J. Montplaisir, R. Godbout, and P. Lavoisier. Sexual activity and sleep in humans. *Biolog. Psych.* 1985; 20:758–63.

Leitenberg, H., and K. Henning. Sexual fantasy. *Psycholog. Bull.* 1994; 117(3):469–96.

Wise, T. N. Difficulty falling asleep after coitus. *Med. Aspects Hum. Sex.* 1981; 15:144.

Chapter 7. Sleeping Single in a Double Bed

Lipman, D. *Snoring A to Zzzzzzzzz.* Portland, OR: Spencer Press, 1996.

Pankhurst, F. P., and J. A. Horne. The influence of bed partners on movement during sleep. *Sleep* 1994; 17:308–15.

Real, T. *I Don't Want to Talk About It: Overcoming the Secret Legacy of Male Depression.* New York: Fireside Books, 1997.

Shepard, J., et al. Bed partners lose an hour of sleep per night due to snoring. *Mayo Clinic Proc.* October 4, 1999.

Chapter 8. The Other Sleepers in the House

Blader, J. C., et al. Sleep problems of elementary school children: A community survey. *Arch. Pediatr. Adolesc. Med.* 1997; 151(5):473–80.

Dahl, R. E. The consequences of insufficient sleep for adolescents. *Phi Delta Kappan* 1999; 354–59.

Ferber, R. *Solve Your Child's Sleep Problems.* New York: Fireside/Simon & Schuster, 1985.

Friman, P. C., et al. The bedtime pass: An approach to bedtime crying and leaving the room. *Arch. Pediatr. Adolesc. Med.* 1999; (153):1027–29.

Guilleminault, C. *Sleep and Its Disorders in Children.* New York: Raven, 1987.

Lee, K. A., G. McEnany, and D. Weeks. Gender differences in sleep patterns for early adolescents. *J. Adolesc. Health* 1999; 24:16–20.

Owens, J., et al. Television viewing habits and sleep disturbance in schoolchildren. *Pediatrics,* 1999; 104(3).

Stein, M. A., et al. Unraveling sleep problems in treated and untreated children with ADHD. *J. Child Adolesc. Psychopharm.* November 1999.

Wahlstrom, K. I. The prickly politics of school starting times. *Phi Delta Kappan,* January 1999, 345–59.

Weitzman, E. D., et al. Delayed sleep phase syndrome: A chronobiological disorder with sleep onset insomnia. *Arch. Gen. Psych.* 1981; 38.

Index